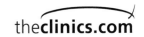

OTOLARYNGOLOGIC CLINICS

OF NORTH AMERICA

Revision Ear and Lateral
Skull Base Surgery

GUEST EDITORS
Richard J. Wiet, MD, FACS
and Robert A. Battista, MD, FACS

August 2006 • Volume 39 • Number 4

SAUNDERS

An Imprint of Elsevier, Inc.
PHILADELPHIA   LONDON   TORONTO   MONTREAL   SYDNEY   TOKYO

W.B. SAUNDERS COMPANY
A Division of Elsevier Inc.

1600 John F. Kennedy Boulevard, Suite 1800, Philadelphia, PA 19103–2899

http://www.theclinics.com

OTOLARYNGOLOGIC CLINICS
OF NORTH AMERICA
August 2006
Editor: Joanne Husovski

Volume 39, Number 4
ISSN 0030–6665
ISBN 1-4160-3925-2

The ideas and opinions expressed in *Otolaryngologic Clinics of North America* do not necessarily reflect those of the Publisher. The Publisher does not assume any responsibility for any injury and/or damage to persons or property arising out of or related to any use of the material contained in this periodical. The reader is advised to check the appropriate medical literature and the product information currently provided by the manufacturer of each drug to be administered to verify the dosage, the method and duration of administration, or contraindications. It is the responsibility of the treating physician or other health care professional, relying on independent experience and knowledge of the patient, to determine drug dosages and the best treatment for the patient. Mention of any product in this issue should not be construed as endorsement by the contributors, editors, or the Publisher of the product or manufacturers' claims.

Otolaryngologic Clinics of North America (ISSN 0030–6665) is published bimonthly by Elsevier Inc., 360 Park Avenue South, New York, NY 10010-1710. Months of issue are February, April, June, August, October, and December. Business and Editorial Offices: 1600 John F. Kennedy Blvd., Suite 1800, Philadelphia, PA 19103-2899. Customer Service Office: 6277 Sea Harbor Drive, Orlando, FL 32887-4800. Periodicals postage paid at New York, NY and additional mailing offices. Subscription price is $205.00 per year (US individuals), $370.00 per year (US institutions), $100.00 per year (US student/resident), $270.00 per year (Canadian individuals), $455.00 per year (Canadian institutions), $285.00 per year (international individuals), $455.00 per year (international institutions), $145.00 per year (international & Canadian student/resident). Foreign air speed delivery is included in all *Clinics'* subscription prices. All prices are subject to change without notice. **POSTMASTER:** Send address changes to *Otolaryngologic Clinics of North America*, Elsevier Periodicals Customer Service, 6277 Sea Harbor Drive, Orlando, FL 32887-4800. **Customer Service: 1-800-654-2452 (US). From outside the US, call 407-345-4000.**

Otolaryngologic Clinics of North America is also published in Spanish by McGraw-Hill Interamericana Editores S.A., P.O. Box 5-237, 06500 Mexico D.F., Mexico.

Otolaryngologic Clinics of North America is covered in *Index Medicus, Current Contents/Clinical Medicine, Excerpta Medica, BIOSIS, Science Citation Index,* and *ISI/BIOMED.*

Printed in the United States of America.

GUEST EDITORS

RICHARD J. WIET, MD, FACS, Professor of Clinical Otolaryngology and Neurosurgery, Northwestern University Feinberg School of Medicine, Chicago, Illinois; Attending Physician, Hinsdale Hospital, Hinsdale, Illinois; Attending Physician, Northwestern Memorial Hospital, Chicago, Illinois; Ear Institute of Chicago, LLC, Hinsdale, Illinois

ROBERT A. BATTISTA, MD, FACS, Assistant Professor of Clinical Otolaryngology, Department of Otolaryngology, Northwestern University Feinberg School of Medicine, Chicago, Illinois; Ear Institute of Chicago, LLC, Hinsdale, Illinois

CONTRIBUTORS

ARLENE BARR, MD, Department of Neurology and Rehabilitation, University of Illinois at Chicago, Chicago, Illinois

ROBERT A. BATTISTA, MD, FACS, Assistant Professor of Clinical Otolaryngology, Department of Otolaryngology, Northwestern University Feinberg School of Medicine, Chicago, Illinois; Ear Institute of Chicago, LLC, Hinsdale, Illinois

NIKOLAS H. BLEVINS, MD, Department of Otolaryngology–Head & Neck Surgery, Stanford University School of Medicine, Stanford, California

IVAN CIRIC, MD, Professor of Neurosurgery, Northwestern University Feinberg School of Medicine, Chicago, Illinois; Chief of Neurosurgery Service, Evanston Northwestern Hospital, Evanston, Illinois

NOEL L. COHEN, MD, Professor of Otolaryngology, Department of Otolaryngology, New York University School of Medicine, New York, New York

GIUSEPPE DE DONATO, MD, Gruppo Otologico, Piacenza, Italy

MAURIZIO FALCIONI, MD, Gruppo Otologico, Piacenza, Italy

J.V.D. HOUGH, MD, Clinical Professor of Otolaryngology, University of Oklahoma Health Sciences Center; Hough Ear Institute, Oklahoma City, Oklahoma

TINA C. HUANG, MD, Neurotology Fellow, Department of Otolaryngology, New York University School of Medicine, New York, New York

ROBERT K. JACKLER, MD, Sewall Professor and Chair, Department of Otolaryngology–Head & Neck Surgery, Stanford University School of Medicine, Stanford, California

JENNIFER JOY, MA, CCC-A, FAAA, Head Clinical Audiologist, Ear Institute of Chicago, LLC, Hinsdale, Illinois

ROBERT P. KAZAN, MD, Director of Neurosciences, Hinsdale Hospital; West Suburban Neurological Associates, Hinsdale, Illinois

ARVIND KUMAR, MD, FRCS, Professor of Otolaryngology, Department of Otolaryngology–Head and Neck Surgery, Department of Neurosurgery, University of Illinois; Adjunct Professor, Department of Otolaryngology Head and Neck Surgery, Northwestern University Feinberg School of Medicine, Chicago, Illinois; Ear Institute of Chicago, LLC, Hinsdale, Illinois

JOHN F. KVETON, MD, Clinical Professor of Surgery/Otolaryngology, Yale University School of Medicine, New Haven, Connecticut

PHILIP D. LITTLEFIELD, MD, Neurotology Fellow, Northwestern University Feinberg School of Medicine, Chicago, Illinois

JOSEPH B. NADOL, JR, MD, Walter Augustus Lecompte Professor and Chairman, Department of Otology and Laryngology, Harvard Medical School; Chief of Otolaryngology, Massachusetts Eye and Ear Infirmary, Boston, Massachusetts

ANH NGUYEN-HUYNH, MD, PhD, Department of Otolaryngology–Head & Neck Surgery, Stanford University School of Medicine, Stanford, California

MICHAEL M. PAPARELLA, MD, Director, Otology/Neurotology Fellowship, Minnesota Ear, Head and Neck Clinic; Director, Otopathology Laboratory, Clinical Professor, and Chairman Emeritus, Department of Otolaryngology, University of Minnesota; International Hearing Foundation, Minneapolis, Minnesota

MYLES L. PENSAK, MD, FACS, Professor and Chairman, The Neuroscience Institute, Department of Otolaryngology, University of Cincinnati/Cincinnati Children's Hospital Medical Center, Cincinnati, Ohio

PAOLO PIAZZA, MD, Department of Neuroradiology, University of Parma, Parma, Italy

J. THOMAS ROLAND, JR, MD, Associate Professor of Otolaryngology and Neurosurgery, Director Otology/Neurotology, Co-director NYU Cochlear Implant Program, Department of Otolaryngology, New York University School of Medicine, New York, New York

JOHN RYZENMAN, MD, Department of Otolaryngology Head and Neck Surgery, Feinberg School of Medicine, Northwestern University, Chicago, Illinois

RAVI N. SAMY, MD, FACS, Assistant Professor, The Neuroscience Institute, Department of Otolaryngology, University of Cincinnati/Cincinnati Children's Hospital Medical Center, Cincinnati, Ohio

MARIO SANNA, MD, Gruppo Otologico, Piacenza, Italy

RICHARD J. WIET, MD, FACS, Professor of Clinical Otolaryngology and Neurosurgery, Northwestern University Feinberg School of Medicine, Chicago, Illinois; Attending Physician, Hinsdale Hospital, Hinsdale, Illinois; Attending Physician, Northwestern Memorial Hospital, Chicago, Illinois; Ear Institute of Chicago, LLC, Hinsdale, Illinois

CONTENTS

Not long ago, the restoration of a perforated tympanic membrane by grafting over an air-containing tympanic cavity seemed impossible. Fortunately, successful results are so consistent and universal today that restoration of the tympanic membrane is expected, and a failure calls for careful evaluation as to "why." If known principles are observed, few complications need occur. Usually, complications are the result of either the choice and placement of the graft used in the repair, or the presence of unresolved upper respiratory pathology. When revision tympanoplasty is necessary, use of the underlay fascial graft technique, properly applied, usually can solve any difficult problems.

Revision stapedectomy can be a technically demanding operation. The surgeon must be prepared for many pathologic conditions before revision stapes surgery. Appropriate preoperative patient counseling is a must. The best chance for hearing improvement is in those cases that have a delayed conductive hearing loss after primary stapedectomy. This article serves as a guideline for discussing the myriad possibilities that may be encountered during this type of revision stapedectomy. Indications for revision stapedectomy and general surgical guidelines for management of specific pathologic conditions are discussed. The material presented is based on literature review, the authors' personal experience, and a review of temporal bone studies relative to stapes surgery.

Revision Ossiculoplasty

Ravi N. Samy and Myles L. Pensak

Although ossiculoplasty, also known as ossicular chain reconstruction (OCR), was attempted initially in the early 1900s, it was not until the 1950s that it became commonplace and relatively well understood. Since then, there have been numerous technologic advances and a gain in the understanding of ossiculoplasty. However, successful OCR with resulting long-term stability can be a daunting task. Typically, the most common condition requiring revision OCR is chronic suppurative otitis media (COM) with or without cholesteatoma. Primary and revision OCR are performed also for blunt and penetrating trauma-induced conductive hearing loss, congenital defects (eg, atresia), and benign and malignant tumors. Typically, reconstruction in ears with COM is more difficult than in ears without infection. This article discusses the key factors involved in successful revision OCR.

Endolymphatic Sac Revision for Recurrent Intractable Meniere's Disease

Michael M. Paparella

Meniere's disease can be observed uniquely in revisions of the conservative surgical procedure for endolymphatic sac enhancement, which preserves the labyrinth, unlike destructive procedures. Genetic anatomic abnormalities in patients lead to malabsorption of endolymph and symptoms of Meniere's that are reversed by endolymphatic sac enhancement, but disabling symptoms eventually may recur in a few cases and require revisional surgery. We observe developing pathophysiologic conditions intraoperatively and have modified our techniques to accommodate the redeveloped pathogenesis we observe and avoid complications found with earlier techniques. This conservative treatment allows patients (many of whom may develop bilateral Meniere's) to retain capacity to accept cochlear implants should they become advisable later.

Revision Mastoidectomy

Joseph B. Nadol Jr.

The first three priorities in surgery for chronic otitis media are (1) the elimination of progressive disease to produce a safe and dry ear, (2) modification of the anatomy of the tympanomastoid compartment to prevent recurrent disease, and (3) reconstruction of the hearing mechanism. The indications for revision following mastoidectomy for chronic otitis media thus involve failure to achieve any of these goals, including recurrent cholesteatoma, recurrent suppuration, recurrent perforation, or recurrent or residual conductive hearing loss. The focus of this article is the management of recurrent cholesteatoma or suppuration; that is, failure to achieve either of the first two priorities.

Revision Surgery for Vertigo

John F. Kveton

When confronted with vertigo after an otologic procedure, a surgeon first must identify the functional status of the inner ear by performing auditory and vestibular testing. Using this information in conjunction with knowledge of the primary disease process for which the initial procedure was performed, the surgeon can make a rational selection of the procedure required to eliminate vertigo. This article outlines a systematic approach to the selection of the appropriate revision procedure and discusses the specific advantages and disadvantages of these procedures used to control vertigo.

Acoustic Neuroma (Vestibular Schwannoma) Revision

Richard J. Wiet, Robert P. Kazan, Ivan Ciric, and Philip D. Littlefield

The authors present their experience of more than 25 years, now in excess of 1200 patients, with cerebellopontine angle tumors. This article focuses on the management of planned subtotal resection of acoustic tumors in five subjects, and unexpected "residual" discovered by MRI scanning in 10 cases, which represents, to the best of the authors' knowledge, a residual rate of 1% of operated patients. The rate of residual tumor is as high as 19% in some series and, in part, depends on the surgical approach. For the purpose of this article, the authors did not include their cases of neurofibromatosis, because these tumors behave differently than unilateral sporadic schwannomas.

Revision Glomus Tumor Surgery

Mario Sanna, Giuseppe De Donato, Paolo Piazza, and Maurizio Falcioni

The infratemporal fossa approach type A is the best way to deal with recurrent tympano-jugular paragangliomas because facial nerve rerouting is fundamental to reaching the area of the internal carotid artery, where recurrence is likely to occur. Preservation of lower cranial nerve function is not feasible when there is tumor infiltration of the medial wall of the jugular bulb; any attempt at nerve dissection increases the risk of leaving some tumor remnants. Correct management of the internal carotid artery, including preoperative stent insertion or permanent preoperative balloon occlusion, is usually a fundamental step when dealing with these highly vascularized lesions. Because of the tumor tendency to infiltrate the bony structures, aggressive drilling of the temporal bone is also advised, especially at the level of the petrous apex. Patients affected by uncontrolled recurrences still die of this disease.

of an existing device with immediate or delayed reimplantation, or for scalp flap revision and receiver-stimulator repositioning in the case of infection or device migration. Rarely, revision surgery is performed to reintroduce intracochlear electrodes that may have partly or entirely extruded from the cochlea or were placed inappropriately. Successful revision cochlear implant surgery requires attention to certain surgical principles. Good outcomes, as measured by speech perception tests, are common, but are not guaranteed. This article outlines the indications for revision cochlear implant surgery, the recommended surgical principles, and published outcomes from reimplantation.

FORTHCOMING ISSUES

RECENT ISSUES

ELSEVIER
SAUNDERS

Otolaryngol Clin N Am
39 (2006) xi–xii

OTOLARYNGOLOGIC
CLINICS
OF NORTH AMERICA

Preface

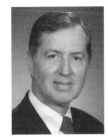 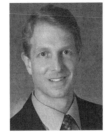

Richard J. Wiet, MD, FACS   Robert A. Battista, MD, FACS
Guest Editors

Since the inception of the *Otolaryngologic Clinics of North America* in 1968, few issues have been devoted to the topic of revision surgery. To our knowledge, only one issue has dealt with revision surgery for ear disease in this nearly 40-year period. It is timely, then that revision surgery be revisited and the topic reviewed.

The authors of this issue were chosen because they are well published and respected for their experience in the field of otology, neurotology, and lateral skull base surgery. They have a minimum life experience of 15 years in the field so that they can share their experience hardened and shaped by time. We are grateful for the very valuable personal time they took to contribute to this issue.

We have the opinion that revision surgery for otology, neurotology and lateral skull base surgery is slowly, but inevitably, increasing. The reasons for this increase are multiple, including the lack of appropriate otology, neurotology and lateral skull base surgery material in otolaryngology training programs. Several recent publications have addressed the issue of the lack of otologic/neurotologic procedures performed in otolaryngology residencies. Another reason for the increase in revision surgery is the reluctance to achieve a mastery of ear surgery, either due to the dexterity demands required in microsurgery; or the relative infrequency of case material for otolaryngology practitioners. In addition, the types of surgical procedures in otology, neurotology, and lateral skull base surgery have expanded. Several conditions that were considered inoperable several years ago are now treated routinely with surgery. With this in mind, it is inevitable that more

0030-6665/06/$ - see front matter © 2006 Elsevier Inc. All rights reserved.
doi:10.1016/j.otc.2006.05.002

oto.theclinics.com

revision cases would develop. And finally, perhaps most significantly, we are facing an exploding growth of an aging population.

We know now that the Baby Boom generation (those born between 1946 and 1964) is approaching age 60. According to the February 2006 Bulletin of the American Academy of Otolaryngology–Head and Neck Surgery, 76 million Americans—28% of the United States population—are included in this demographic. A recent *Wall Street Journal* report states that 1 American is now turning 65 every 7 seconds. It is inevitable that, in the case of individuals with a chronic disease, we will have the continued need to hone our skills in revision surgery.

It is our hope that the reader will find this issue of revision ear and lateral skull base surgery of immense value, and we again thank our contributors to this issue.

Richard J. Wiet, MD, FACS
Robert A. Battista, MD, FACS
Department of Otolaryngology–Head and Neck Surgery
Northwestern University Feinberg School of Medicine
Chicago, IL, USA
and
Ear Institute of Chicago, LLC
950 N. York Road, Suite 102
Hinsdale, IL 60521, USA

E-mail addresses:
r-wiet@northwestern.edu
r-battista2@northwestern.edu

**ELSEVIER
SAUNDERS**

Otolaryngol Clin N Am
39 (2006) xiii

OTOLARYNGOLOGIC
CLINICS
OF NORTH AMERICA

Dedication

To our wives, Jamee and Tracy, for all of the support they have given—for they are the *best* part of our daily lives.

Richard J. Wiet, MD, FACS
Robert A. Battista, MD, FACS

0030-6665/06/$ - see front matter © 2006 Elsevier Inc. All rights reserved.
doi:10.1016/j.otc.2006.07.001   *oto.theclinics.com*

ELSEVIER
SAUNDERS

Otolaryngol Clin N Am
39 (2006) 661–675

OTOLARYNGOLOGIC
CLINICS
OF NORTH AMERICA

Revision Tympanoplasty Including Anterior Perforations and Lateralization of Grafts

J.V.D. Hough, MD

Hough Ear Institute, 3400 NW 56th Street, Oklahoma City, OK 73112-4463, USA

Not long ago, the restoration of a perforated tympanic membrane by grafting over an air-containing tympanic cavity seemed impossible. Fortunately, successful results are so consistent and universal today that restoration of the tympanic membrane is expected, and a failure calls for careful evaluation as to "why." This article addresses some of the most common reasons for success or failure in tympanoplasty and describes how to correct the failures.

Common causes of tympanoplastic failure

The most common causes of tympanoplastic failure are

- Unresolved upper respiratory pathology
- Choice of surgical procedure
- Choice of tissue used in grafting
- Postoperative trapped epithelial seed cells
- Use of lateral grafting technique (onlay)

The purpose of this article is to uncover the causes of tympanoplastic failure and offer a surgical restoration technique (revision tympanoplasty).

Choice of surgical procedures

Clinical evaluation of both the patient in general and the site in particular is obviously the first important step. Emphasis on the patient's general health, with specific microscopic study of the ear, and on obtaining full

E-mail address: jhough@houghearinstitute.com

knowledge of the events before, during, and after the previous surgery is crucial. Knowledge of the techniques used previously is the information base for corrective surgery.

Since modern tympanoplastic procedures were introduced, two distinct techniques have emerged [1]. Although both techniques have numerous similarities and have produced high rates of success [1,2], they differ in terms of major issues, including their titles (ie, "underlay" versus "onlay," or "medial graft tympanoplasty" versus "lateral graft tympanoplasty.")

The underlay or medial graft technique usually uses fascia from the lateral surface of the temporalis muscle, whereas the onlay or lateral graft technique uses skin grafts on the lateral surface of the drum remnant and canal wall. Because both techniques reportedly give excellent results, these dissimilarities would seem to be of no consequence.

However, since the fascial graft underlay or medial graft technique was introduced, its advantages over other methods, including the onlay graft technique, have been consistent [2]. Since then, it has become the most commonly used surgical approach to correcting pathology and functional deficits in both primary and revision tympanoplasty.

Therefore, in this article, the specific repair of three of the more common postoperative complications, lateralization of the tympanic membrane from the handle of the malleus, reperforation of the anterior drumhead, and pullaway from the handle of the malleus, are all approached using the basic underlay technique. The usual primary underlay surgical procedure is described first, followed by a description of its application to the revision of the above complications.

Primary underlay graft technique

The identifying cardinal principles of the underlay technique, elegantly simple and immediately explanatory, are summarized as follows:

Temporalis fascial grafts are placed first under the tympanic membrane remnant; second, under the handle of the malleus; third, under the anterior annular ligament of the entire tympanic membrane remnant; and fourth, under the canal tympanomeatal skin flap [2]. All normal squamous epithelium remaining on the tympanic membrane remnant is preserved so that the circumferential growth of squamous epithelial cells around the edges of the perforation can cover the defect produced by the perforation rapidly. Skin is not removed from the ear canal. This squamous epithelium is not disturbed over the annular ligament or in the depths of the sulcus, simply because the graft itself is placed underneath these structures and can obtain its blood supply from the mucous membrane in the middle ear, preventing lateralization of the graft, blunting of the anterior angle, and the tendency toward atresia. The only visualization of the tympanic membrane remnant required with the underlay technique is the edge of the perforation anteriorly [1,2].

Surgical technique

Anesthesia

In adults and older cooperative children, approximately 1cc of a local anesthetic with 1% lidocaine and adrenaline is injected into the ear canal. Secondly, a scalp incision above the external ear is injected with approximately 5cc of 1% lidocaine and adrenaline. The external ear canal and surrounding scalp are sterilized with Betadine solution, using extreme care not to allow the solution to drip through the perforation into the middle ear.

Exposure

The principal aim of exposure is to be able to see the entire rim of the tympanic membrane perforation through the speculum in the ear canal. However, it is not necessary to see all areas simultaneously. Different areas of the ear can be seen by manipulating the table, the head of the patient, and so forth. In approximately 10% of ears, the anterior bulge of the exterior ear canal obscures visualization of the entire anterior perforation, the anterior sulcus, and the annular ligament (Fig. 1) [1,3]. Initially, this situation might appear to require a postauricular incision to obtain a view of the depth of the anterior sulcus. Indeed, the onlay technique requires complete removal of all squamous epithelium from the entire outer surface of the drumhead, the entire annular ligament, and the most inaccessible anterior sulcus. However, if the underlay technique is used, the squamous epithelial over the tympanic membrane is a "friend" to the more rapid healing process. It is therefore not necessary to see the entire drum remnant. Only the rim of the perforation needs to be visualized, not the depths of the anterior sulcus.

If the edge of the anterior remnant cannot be seen properly, a Wright-Guilford flap is raised from over the bulge of the anterior canal wall (see Fig. 1) [1]. To do this, an incision is made circumferentially with a Rosen

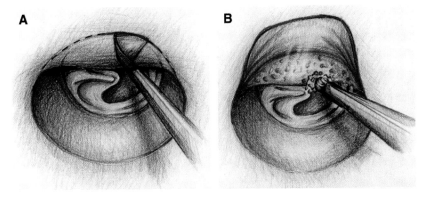

Fig. 1. (A) Anterior canal bulge preventing visualization of the anterior tympanic membrane. (B) Removal of the bony bulge with a diamond burr.

knife, approximately 7 mm lateral to the tympanic membrane. An incision starting at each end of this incision is then made laterally. The skin and periosteum are elevated from the bony hump, laterally exposing the bone. The anterior bony niche and the annular ligament are not disturbed. Often, by removing the thickness of the skin of the anterior canal wall, proper visualization of the anterior tympanic membrane is obtained. If not, enough bone may be removed with a diamond drill burr to permit visualization of the rim of the perforation. It is not necessary to remove bone to the extent that the depths of the sulcus can be visualized. Even in the 10% of cases requiring increased exposure, the amount of surgery required to provide the exposure is far less than the extensive soft tissue dissection and bone drilling necessary in the postauricular approach. After drum reconstruction, the anterior canal wall skin is replaced over the bone.

Preparation of the tympanic membrane remnant for grafting

The temporalis fascial graft is placed in the tympanic cavity medial to the tympanic membrane remnant [1] and the tympanomeatal flap. Its bed on the undersurface of the tympanic membrane remnant should be prepared by delicately denuding mucous membrane from under the surface of the drum remnant [2], by using a "drum scraper" instrument (Fig. 2). With this instrument extending under the remnant of the drum for 1 to 5 mm, engaging the claw tip in the mucous membrane and pulling it toward the edge of the perforation, the mucous membrane is everted toward the perforation

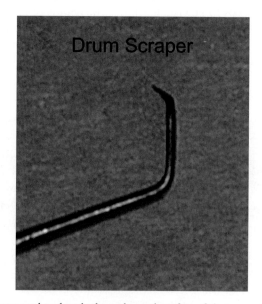

Fig. 2. Drum scraper used to denude the underneath surface of the tympanic membrane remnant during the underlay fascial graft tympanoplasty technique.

and removed. This procedure should be done even in the deep bony niche medial to the annular ligament and even extending down the lateral wall of the eustachian tube. This undersurface preparation should be done in all areas of the hypotympanic recess and drum remnant. This partial mucous membrane removal produces a raw vascular bed to nourish the graft.

After everting the mucous membrane epithelium from under the tympanic membrane and around the perforation, the margin of the perforation is made raw to stimulate epithelial regrowth for a natural closure of the perforation over the underlying fascial graft, accomplished by making pick holes around the circumferential edge of the perforation and joining them with a pick (Fig. 3A) [2]. After this, the collar of the squamous epithelium around the edge of the perforation is removed with cup forceps, allowing an open door for epithelial cells to grow over the fascia and close the perforation (Fig. 3B).

Removal of secondary pathology of the tympanic membrane

Although this disease is not progressive, large tympanosclerotic plaques in the remaining tympanic membrane remnant that impede hearing should be removed, especially when the plaques are in the upper quadrants of the drumhead and cause restricted motion. If a plaque reaches a circumferential edge of the tympanic membrane, attaches to the handle of the malleus, or is thick and well formed, it should be removed. Frequently, the plaque can be fractured inward and removed piecemeal. Often, plaques can be dissected from the medial surface of the squamous epithelial covering without destroying the important squamous epithelial surfaces. Even though this leaves a very thin epithelial layer, any squamous epithelial cells that can be placed over the fascial graft will permit more rapid coverage in the healing process.

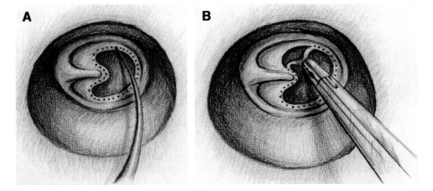

Fig. 3. (*A*) Circumferential pick holes through the mucous membrane around the rim of the tympanic membrane perforation. (*B*) Cup forceps removing the rim of the epithelium around the perforation.

Pathology in the tympanic cavity

After the above is accomplished, the surgeon is prepared to surgically enter, evaluate, and correct related middle ear pathology, through a transcanal Rosen-type incision. This routine stapedectomy incision, approximately 6 to 8 mm lateral to the tympanic membrane, is made in the posterior-superior canal skin, which is elevated. The annular ring is lifted out of its sulcus, exposing the posterior half of the tympanic cavity. If the incudostapedial joint and the mucous membrane extending into the epitympanum cannot be seen sufficiently, the surgeon may remove bone from the posterior-superior bony canal rim. The area of the stapes, incus, and mucous membrane extending into the epitympanum is the tympanomastoid expressway for pathologic entry into the mastoid complex (Fig. 4) [1–3]. If the surgeon can visualize the epitympanum in this area and it is clear, then no further exploration is necessary. However, if cholesteatoma is present or the mucous membrane indicates pathologic tissue, further exposure of the complete middle ear mastoid complex can be obtained easily for complete surgical management, through extension of the original incision laterally by converting it to an endaural incision. All other pathologic problems found in the tympanic cavity and the adnexa can be addressed through this transcanal approach.

In some cases, tympanosclerotic plaques are seen subepithelially in the mucous membrane of the tympanic membrane cavity. If so, the plaques can be peeled away carefully from the outer squamous epithelial surface, but only with extreme delicacy around the crura of the stapes.

The most common areas of involvement in order of occurrence are in the stapedius tendon, along the inferior side of the oval window, around the

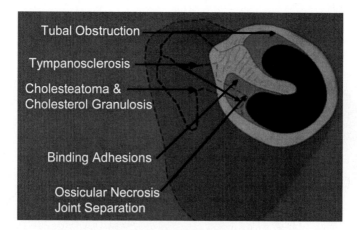

Fig. 4. Tympanomastoid expressway for pathologic entry into the mastoid complex. (*From* Highlights of the Instructional Courses, Volume VI, 1994, edited by Frank Lucente, MD, "Tympanoplasty-Reconstruction of the Tympanic Membrane," Hough JVD, Baker RS, Mosby Year Book, Vol. 7, 28:307–13, 1995; with permission.)

round window niche, and along the facial nerve [2]. Normally, if no further inflammatory activity is present, these plaques do not regrow.

Other troublesome problems that need repair may also be present, such as congential deformities, ossicular necrosis, or fractures and dislocations [1,2]. Many of these problems can be repaired successfully at the time of the original surgery and does not always require a secondary procedure.

Obtaining the temporalis fascial graft

To obtain the temporalis fascial graft [4,5], an incision of approximately 2 cm long is made above the external ear and dissection is carried down to the superficial layer of the temporalis fascia. The soft tissues are elevated from the lateral surface of the fascia with an elevator over an area measuring approximately 4 to 5 cm. A small incision is then made horizontally at the inferior edge of the exposed fascia. With the elevator, the fascia is dissected from the lateral surface of the temporalis muscle. With Foman upper lateral cartilage scissors (Fig. 5), the graft, measuring approximately 2.5 cm by 3 cm, is then removed. The wound is closed with interrupted sutures.

The graft should not be allowed to dry out or be compressed. If not used immediately, it can be placed in a moisturized tissue bath consisting of a Petrie dish containing three or four moist cotton balls.

When ready to use, the fascia is placed on a Teflon disc and excessive connective tissue is removed. The graft is then trimmed so that when placed, the entire tympanic cavity will be covered and there is an extension of tissue to cover the bone from which the tympanomeatal flap has been elevated (Fig. 6A) [2]. Gelfoam (Upjohn, Kalamazoo, Michigan) is then pressed in the package with a Gelfoam press, removed from the package, and cut to fit a portion of the graft the size of the tympanic cavity (see Fig. 6A). The Gelfoam is placed on the inferior surface of the fascia to be used as a plate to guide the fascia under the tympanomeatal flap into the middle ear. The

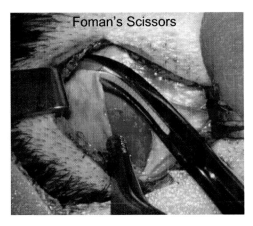

Fig. 5. Removal of temporalis fascia with Foman upper lateral scissors.

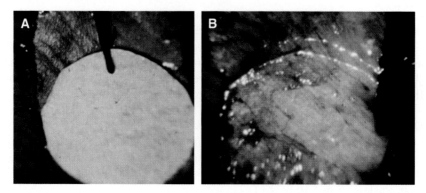

Fig. 6. (*A*) Temporalis fascia graft with Gelfoam disc. (*B*) Gelfoam disc placed under the fascial graft ready for insertion.

graft, with its absorbable Gelfoam backing, is picked up with cup forceps on its anterior margin and inserted into the tympanic cavity so that the Gelfoam provides a middle ear bed for the new tympanic membrane.

Graft insertion

The graft is moved under the tympanomeatal flap, under the handle of the malleus, and under the annular ligament both anteriorly and posteriorly. The anterior placement of the graft is the key to its success.

I have found the use of two instruments to be very helpful [6]. The Derlacki mobilizer tucks the edges of the graft into place and the Cadogan foot-pedal–controlled suction (Cadogan Manufacturing, Oklahoma City, Oklahoma) (Fig. 7) keeps the operative site clean and is useful in moving Gelfoam and tissues around and releasing them with precision.

After the graft is guided under the handle of the malleus with a Derlacki mobilizer and foot pedal suction, it is moved forward to the anterior tympanic cavity with cup forceps, a Derlacki mobilizer, and foot pedal suction.

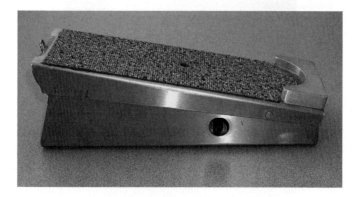

Fig. 7. Cadogan foot-pedal–controlled suction.

It is spread out anteriorly until it is completely under the anterior annular ligament and is filling the anterior recesses of the tympanic cavity. When the graft has been moved anteriorly enough so that its trailing edge covers the bone in the posterior canal wall, instrumentation is used to smooth it out so that it completely covers the exposed bone of the posterior canal wall and meets the original tympanomeatal flap canal incision.

After the graft has been positioned over the posterior bony canal wall and the tympanomeatal flap has been returned to its normal position, attention is turned to the vital areas of the anterior sulcus. The graft is approached anteriorly through the perforation and is moved forward to completely fill the anterior middle ear cavity and under the anterior annular ligament.

Superiorly, in the area of the eustachian tube, is the deepest portion of the middle ear and frequently the graft will retract or fall into the deeper space. The graft and the Gelfoam can be rolled back out with cup forceps to expose the eustachian tube area and the depth of the sulcus. Wet Gelfoam is then placed in these areas until the graft can be replaced so that it fits snugly under the annular ligament and deep into the recesses of the anterior tympanic cavity. It is also good to place Gelfoam a short distance down the eustachian tube to hold the graft on its lateral surface.

A final inspection of the vital anterior sulcus areas is made to ensure that the graft is closing the tympanic membrane perforation totally. With controlled suction, the area can be cleared of tissue fluids without a danger of moving the graft accidentally after it has been placed carefully. If the anterior Wright-Guilford flap was made to reduce the anterior bulge of the canal wall, this flap is then returned to its normal position. Wet Gelfoam pledgets are helpful in not only providing the nutrition and base for the graft, but also in holding it in position. Lastly, after the graft is in good position, Gelfoam is placed on the lateral side of the graft, filling the ear canal and ending the primary underlay fascial graft surgical procedure.

The procedure of primary underlay fascial graft tympanoplasty has been described, showing the principles of this surgery and the postoperative results that guide the selection of this procedure. When failures occur, this same logical technique is used with special accommodation added, which is described as each problem of revision tympanoplasty is approached.

Revision tympanoplasty

The title "Revision tympanoplasty" directs attention to three major complications that plague surgeons and patients after failed tympanoplasty: pull-away from the handle of the malleus, blunting of the anterior angle, and reperforation of the tympanic membrane. These disappointing results can be explained and often corrected. However, with the proper primary technique they probably can be prevented. Understanding the natural function of the external ear canal and tympanic membrane, and the response to tissues used in the repair of defects, is as important as past experience.

A straightforward critique of inadequate surgical approaches and poor decision-making decisions regarding known tissue responses is made, along with a discussion on correct surgical technique and grafting materials [2,4,5].

Pull-away from the handle of the malleus

Part of the reason for this mysterious complication (Fig. 8) is thought to be the powerful pull of the migratory activity of the skin's squamous epithelium. The ear canal cleanses itself through the constant movement and desquamation of the outer layers of the squamous epithelial cells of the medial ear canal moving toward the exterior. Therefore, if a skin graft is placed on the lateral surface of the handle of the malleus, it becomes vulnerable to being enveloped in this lateral force (Fig. 9).

To manage this physiologic force properly, the fascial graft should be placed under the handle of the malleus, as in the underlay technique [2]. This step prevents lateralization and provides an anchor to hold the graft in position. If this principle has not been observed in the original surgical procedure and there is a pull-away from the handle of the malleus requiring revision of the tympanoplasty, the problem is solved by going back to correct the original mistake. In other words, after removing the lateralized tympanic membrane and dissecting the graft from the lateral surface of the tympanic membrane remnant, the usual procedure for the underlay fascial graft technique is performed.

Revision surgery

More specifically, to correct this, the tympanic membrane and tympanomeatal flap are elevated, exposing the tympanic cavity. If the drum is well attached to the anterior annular ligament and there is no anterior blunting, then the only concern is in the region of the handle of the malleus. Another incision is made along the posterior side of the handle of the malleus. The

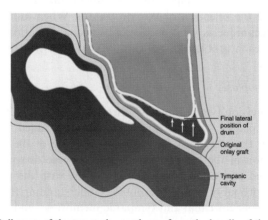

Fig. 8. Pull-away of the tympanic membrane from the handle of the malleus.

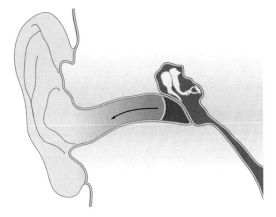

Fig. 9. Migratory pull of squamous epithelium over the tympanic membrane.

skin, soft tissue, and mucous membrane of the malleus are dissected from
the bone, creating an incision over the malleus through the tympanic membrane the length of the handle of the malleus in the center of the tympanic
membrane. A small strip of temporalis fascia is then obtained, thinned, and
cut to fit the defect. The fascia is draped under the handle of the malleus to
surround the posterior surface of the handle of the malleus, forming a sling.
The arms of the sling are draped around the handle of the malleus and extended through the perforation to loop over the lateral surface of the drumhead, closing the perforation and forming the connecting link of the drum to
the handle of the malleus. All soft tissue is removed from the malleus so that
the raw edges of the perforation can unite with the fascial graft, ensuring
a firm adherence of the tympanic membrane to the handle of the malleus,
upon healing.

If lateralization of the tympanic membrane is a significant distance from
the handle of the malleus and there is blunting of the anterior angle, the defect may be more than a separation of the drumhead from the handle of
the malleus. It may become a lateral atresia of the drum surface toward
the isthmus of the external ear canal, requiring more extensive reconstruction techniques, as described later.

Blunting of the anterior angle of the tympanic membrane

This complication to tympanoplastic surgery (Fig. 10) emphasizes the importance of anatomic and physiologic factors. It is important to keep the entire canal skin intact in order to completely cover the depths of the anterior
sulcus, the anterior annular ligament, and the anterior remnant of the tympanic membrane. If the outer squamous epithelium is removed for the onlay
grafting technique, two disappointing postoperative complications may occur: tympanic membrane pull-away from the handle of the malleus, as discussed earlier, and blunting of the angle.

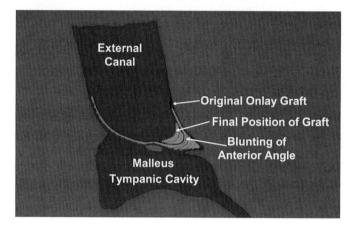

Fig. 10. Anterior blunting of the tympanic membrane. (*From* Highlights of the Instructional Courses, Volume VI, 1994, edited by Frank Lucente, MD, "Tympanoplasty-Reconstruction of the Tympanic Membrane," Hough JVD, Baker RS, Mosby Year Book, Vol. 7, 28:307–13, 1995; with permission.)

An attempt to revise this complication produced by the onlay technique is difficult because the angle at the juncture of the tympanic membrane and anterior canal wall is acute. The thickness of the skin graft overfills the acute angle, causing scarring and blunting. Furthermore, a principle in all healing is to recognize that a graft will round off an acute angle, in this case filling in the bony niche and splinting the anterior tympanic membrane, which can be disabling to the vibratory capacity of the anterior tympanic membrane extending to the handle of the malleus.

In addition, the original removal of the squamous epithelium in this area, together with the removal of the soft tissue that has caused the blunting, will produce this condition again because of the same tendency toward rounding off occurring during the healing process. Nevertheless, revision with the underlay technique can often bring success.

The procedure for revision should be to remove the skin, connective tissue, and mucous membrane in the area of the blunting, and to regraft, which can be done by incorporating this removal and reconstruction with the underlay fascial grafting technique.

Revision surgery

Assuming the blunting extends posteriorly and causes splinting of the handle of the malleus, the procedure could be as follows:

An incision is made at the lateral end of the scar tissue on the anterior canal wall, usually a few millimeters lateral to the annular ligament, down to the bone. An incision is made on both ends of this, down to the annular ligament. The skin of the soft tissue is reflected medially to expose the annular ligament. If the external ear canal is not large enough in diameter for proper instrumentation, the incisions should be extended laterally to produce a Lempert endaural incision with the benefit of wider exposure.

A diamond burr should be used to improve visualization of the annular ligament and anterior bony angle, so that a thorough cleansing of the anterior sulcus can be obtained and to provide a wider angle with a better chance of healing without blunting.

Another incision is made anterior to the handle of the malleus and on either end anteriorly, to connect with the above-mentioned incisions. This block of tissue, which would encompass most of the anterior tympanic membrane, is then removed. A stapedectomy-type incision is then made. The tympanomeatal flap is elevated, and the posterior tympanic membrane with its annular ligament is reflected anteriorly. Mucous membrane excoriation to prepare the graft bed is performed as described in the primary underlay medial graft procedure.

The temporalis fascial graft is removed from the temporalis muscle, placed on a Gelfoam bed as previously described, and placed under the handle of the malleus, under the tympanic membrane remnant, and extended out on the posterior canal wall. The fascial graft is moved forward until it is securely under the anterior annular ligament, into the anterior recess of the tympanic cavity, and into the eustachian tube orifice on its lateral surface. The surface of the fascial graft, which now constitutes the anterior tympanic membrane, is now covered externally with canal wall skin.

The canal wall skin is obtained by making incisions in the anterior canal wall (Wright-Guilford incisions); a generous area of this skin is used as a sliding graft to cover the anterior angle completely and to extend posteriorly to the handle of the malleus. The area is then covered with strips of lubricated Owens cloth and tightly packed, particularly at the angle, with long-fiber small cotton balls. The primary procedure is then followed to its conclusion.

Reperforation of the tympanic membrane anteriorly

The most common failure in tympanoplasty for perforation of the tympanic membrane is reperforation of the new tympanic membrane in the anterior portion. The ear canal is a small tube turned in such a way that the anterior canal wall frequently bulges over, and with a twist in the canal the anterior portion of the eardrum is frequently not seen when looking straight into the ear canal through a speculum. Therefore, many surgeons do not attempt to approach the ear through the canal but resort to needlessly invasive postauricular incisions in the ear canal, removal of bone, and retraction of the soft tissues anteriorly. Unfortunately, this approach often leads to reperforation, caused by either improper repair due to lack of visualization, use of lateral or onlay grafting, recurrence of otitis media, or surgical error in this difficult area that requires delicacy and skill because of the anatomy of the anterior area of the drumhead.

Revision surgery

Reperforation with blunting. If there is blunting of the anterior angle and re-perforation from previous surgery, the techniques for both reperforation and blunting of the anterior angle require the same operative exposure as described previously under "Blunting."

In the case of blunting of the anterior angle, removal of all scar tissue and excessive growth of the angle is necessary. Usually, a Wright-Guilford flap is elevated and bone removed from this area to expose the angle. It is neces-sary to remove the squamous epithelium because of the blunting. Therefore, the canal wall skin must be used in such a way as to recreate an angle to cover the tympanic membrane defect. Because the canal wall skin to be used should be very thin and full thickness, skin from the floor of the canal or anterior canal wall is best for this purpose. The Wright-Guilford skin flap can be used as a sliding graft over the defect anteriorly. The skin graft should be elevated and removed immediately at the time of the incision. Otherwise, tearing of the graft during surgical manipulation often occurs. Orientation as to the lateral or medial end of the graft should be observed carefully.

In grafting the external surface of the tympanic membrane over the un-derlying fascia, it is also important to place the fascia on the medial surface of the drum remnant, extending it far anteriorly under the anterior sulcus and deep on the lateral surface of the orifice of the eustachian tube.

Reperforation without blunting or atresia. The key to the complexity of the surgery required to correct this defect is the presence or absence of the an-nular ligament and the ability to see the circumferential edge of the perfora-tion. If previous surgical procedures have left normal epithelial surfaces covering the normal annular ligament and the edge of the perforation is vis-ible, allowing removal of a very small amount of the epithelial rim of the perforation, the chance of surgical success is greatly improved. In this situ-ation, which is the most common occurrence, the straightforward, classic underlay fascial graft tympanoplasty technique can be done, as described earlier.

Frequently, reperforation can be a simple opening in the tympanic membrane at the edge of the annular ligament with distinct edges as de-scribed. This postoperative complication is caused by inadequate place-ment of grafts, either onlay or underlay, at the time of the primary surgery. Surgical reconstruction is accomplished by applying the underlay tympanoplasty as described and being very careful to place the fascial graft fully in the tympanic cavity recess anteriorly, with great care as to its placement in the deep eustachian tube area. The fascia must cover the me-dial surface of the annular ligament and the tympanic membrane remnant completely, including the posterior tympanic membrane and the tympano-meatal flap.

Summary

If the procedures for reconstruction of the tympanic membrane using the underlay fascial graft technique are followed correctly, three of the more common tympanoplastic complications should not occur. The pull-away of the tympanic membrane from the handle of the malleus is prevented by anchoring the graft under the handle of the malleus. Anterior perforation does not occur because the anterior skin of the ear canal and the annular ligament become the frontier of growth for the new tympanic membrane over the underlay fascial graft. Blunting of the anterior angle does not occur because the anterior angle is not surgically invaded, thus preventing the natural rounding of the corner by onlay grafts and build-up of scar tissue caused by excessive healing in the corner of the anterior sulcus.

References

[1] Glasscock ME. Tympanic membrane grafting with fascia: overlay vs undersurface technique. Laryngoscope 1973;83:754–70.
[2] Hough JVD. Tympanoplasty with interior fascial graft technique and ossicular reconstruction. Laryngoscope 1970;80(9):1385–413.
[3] Austin DF. Transcanal tympanoplasty. Otolaryngol Clin North Am 1972;5(1):127–43.
[4] Storrs LA. Myringoplasty with use of fascia grafts. Arch Otolaryngol 1961;74:45–9.
[5] Ortegren U. Myringoplasty. Four years' experience of temporal fascia grafts. Acta Otolaryngol Suppl 1964;193:1–43.
[6] Hough JVD. Suction control with a foot pedal. Trans Am Acad Ophthalmol Otolaryngol 1966;70:846.

OTOLARYNGOLOGIC
CLINICS
OF NORTH AMERICA

Otolaryngol Clin N Am
39 (2006) 677–697

Revision Stapedectomy

Robert A. Battista, MD, FACS[a,b,*],
Richard J. Wiet, MD, FACS[a,b],
Jennifer Joy, MA, CCC-A, FAAA[b]

[a]Department of Otolaryngology, Northwestern University Feinberg School of Medicine,
12-561 303 E. Chicago Avenue, Chicago, IL 60611, USA
[b]Ear Institute of Chicago, LLC, 950 North York Road, Suite 102, Hinsdale, IL 60521, USA

Stapedectomy surgery was revived by John Shea [1] in 1956 when he developed an appropriate prosthesis. Credit must also be given to Rodney Perkins who developed laser ear surgery, improving the success of revision stapedectomy.

The number of stapes revision cases is rising because of various reasons, such as the decreasing number of stapes surgery available for graduating residents. In 2004, Meyer and Lambert [2] estimated that, over a 6- to 20-year period of observation, 10% to 20% of stapedectomy patients would have a revision to correct for further conductive hearing loss. It is possible that as the population ages, thousands may need revision stapedectomy.

The authors' group has been performing revision stapedectomy for 25 years, and is involved with fellowship and resident education at Northwestern University. The two senior authors share their collective experience in this area. This article focuses on key factors that have led to success, but also includes those cases that are less likely to be successful. The material presented is based on literature review, personal experience, and a review of temporal bone studies relative to stapes surgery.

Primary stapedectomy

Whether a primary or a revision case, the minimum air-bone gap (ABG) requiring surgery should be 20 dB, averaged over the key speech frequencies of 0.5, 1, and 2 kHz. Bilateral conductive loss patients are usually most pleased with a hearing gain in one ear; the authors perform surgery on the second ear

---

* Corresponding author. Ear Institute of Chicago, LLC, 950 North York Road, Suite 102, Hinsdale, IL 60521.

E-mail address: r-battista2@northwestern.edu (R.A. Battista).

doi:10.1016/j.otc.2006.04.003
oto.theclinics.com

only if there were no complications with the first surgery. The surgeon who performs primary stapes surgery must be prepared for surprises in the diagnosis, which could include congenital cholesteatoma, ossicular erosion, tympanosclerosis, and the occasional cerebrospinal fluid (CSF) gusher. An even wider array of pathology is potentially present in revision surgery.

In 1995, the American Academy of Otolaryngology–Head and Neck Surgery Committee on Hearing and Equilibrium [3] provided reporting guidelines for stapes surgery. The ABG is determined by subtracting the postoperative bone pure-tone average (PTA) from the postoperative air PTA. PTA is the four-tone average of 0.5, 1, 2, and 3 kHz. The Committee recommends reporting the mean, standard deviation, and range of the postoperative ABG, and the number of decibels of change. A successful hearing outcome is defined as a postoperative air conduction PTA within 10 dB of the postoperative bone conduction PTA for both primary and revision procedures.

Expected hearing outcomes for revision stapedectomy

The hearing results after revision stapes surgery are generally poorer than those obtained at primary surgery for hearing restoration. Successful hearing results (PTA $\leq$ 10 dB) for revision stapedectomy range from 16% to 80% (mean 53%) (Table 1). The variability in hearing results is due, in part, to the indication for revision. Most of the studies listed in Table 1 report hearing results for a wide range of indications, including conductive hearing loss, dizziness, and suspected perilymphatic fistula (PLF). Successful hearing results are somewhat better (range 40%–80%; mean 57%) (see Table 1) when the indications for revision stapedectomy are confined to persistent or recurrent conductive or mixed hearing loss. Success of up to 91% (N = 35) has been reported when the indication for revision was conductive or mixed hearing loss and a laser was used [4].

Hearing results also depend on the number of revisions. Successful hearing outcomes decrease as revisions increase [4–13]. Most of the studies listed in Table 1 include hearing results for multiple revisions, which may also account for the variable hearing results.

Finally, the risk of sensorineural hearing loss is higher in revision stapedectomy than in the primary case. Sensorineural loss after revision ranges from 0% to 20% (mean 4.5%), with deafness ranging from 0% to 14% (mean 1.7%) (see Table 1).

Indications for revision stapedectomy

Preoperative indications for stapes revisions are categorized generally into one of five areas:

• Conductive hearing loss (delayed or persistent)

Table 1
Literature review: hearing results[a]

Author (year)	N	<10 dB (%)	<20 dB (%)	SNHL (%)	Deaf (%)
Feldman (1970) [10]	142	49	71[c]	0.4	0
Crabtree (1980) [8]	35	46	—	20	14
Lippy (1980) [25][b]	63	49	54	11	—
Sheehy (1981) [7]	258	44	71	7	3.3
Pearman (1982) [56][b]	74	52	66	3	—
Lippy (1983) [63]	100	71	84.5	0	0
Derlacki (1985) [18]	217	60	72	4	1.4
Glasscock (1987) [6]	79	39	64	3	1.2
Bhardwaj (1988) [14]	100	44[c]	—	12	2
Lesinski (1989) [77] (CO_2)[b,d,f]	59	66	87	0	0
Silverstein (1989)[d]	18	66	89	—	—
Farrior (1991) [13]	102	57	84	—	—
Vartiainen (1992) [29][b]	45	45.5	71	4.4	2.2
Prasad (1993) [27][b,g]	41	46	78	12.1	—
McGee (1993) [78] (KTP)[f]	77	80.5	92	2.3	0
Langman (1993) [23]	66	61	84	3	0
Horn (1994) [21] (Argon)[b,f]	32	75	90	0	0
Cokkeser (1994) [15]	49	16	59	—	4
Silverstein (1994) [79]	24	37.5	50	—	—
Silverstein (1994) [79] (Argon/KTP)[f]	37	51	70	—	—
Glasscock (1995) [80]	166	68	—	—	2.7
Haberkamp (1996) [19] (CO_2)[b,f]	25	65	76	—	—
Pedersen (1996) [72][b]	163	51	75	1.2	1.6
Han (1997) [5]	60	52	82	4.1	1.3[i]
Wiet (1997) [81] (Argon)[f]	23	52	70	0	0
Magliulo (1997) [82][e]	63	24	59	—	3.1
Somers (1997) [11][b]	226	40	64	3	0
Nissen (1998) [83] (Argon)[b,f,g]	21	43	62	1	0
Hammerschlag (1998) [20][b,d,h]	250	80	85[a]	2	0
De La Cruz (2000) [17] (Argon/CO_2)[f,g]	356	59.8	77.5	7.7	1.4
Lippy (2003) [4][b]	483	71	86.3	2	1
Gros (2005)[g]	63	52.4	79.4	—	1

Abbreviations: N, number of cases in the study; SNHL, sensorineural hearing loss; —, no data recorded.

[a] Postoperative air minus preoperative bone conduction pure-tone average at 0.5, 1, 2 kHz, unless otherwise noted.

[b] Indication for revision confined to persistent or recurrent mixed hearing loss and cases of stapes mobilization at primary surgery excluded.

[c] Gap closure to within 15 dB.

[d] Including frequency 3 kHz.

[e] Including frequency 4 kHz.

[f] With laser. (Type of laser)

[g] Using postoperative air minus postoperative bone at four frequencies.

[h] Using postoperative air minus postoperative bone at three frequencies.

[i] Delayed sudden sensorineural hearing loss after 13 months of hearing improvement.

- Dizziness
- Sensorineural hearing loss
- Distortion of sound
- Other tympanic/middle ear problems (ie, tympanic adhesions, perforations, cholesteatoma, and so forth)

The opportunity for successful hearing improvement is greatest in cases of delayed conductive hearing loss [4–29]. When revision is performed for conductive hearing loss, it is recommend that the PTA ABG be 20 dB or greater. Revision surgery should be delayed for 6 weeks after the original procedure when a tissue seal (eg, vein, perichondrium, fascia, and so forth) has been used over the oval window [4,30] because the seal causes a localized reaction that would obscure crucial areas of the middle ear.

Delayed conductive hearing loss

By far, the most common indication for revision is delayed (recurrent) conductive hearing impairment [4–29]. The most common reason for a recurrent conductive loss is a displaced prosthesis (Table 2). Several factors may

Table 2
Literature review: intraoperative findings [4–6, 8–11,13–16,18,20,25–27,29,30,47,72,78,82,84–86]

Intraoperative findings	
Prosthesis	N = 3280 (%)
Displaced (from distal or incus)	1192 (36.3)
Short	209 (6.4)
Long	68 (2.1)
Loose	142 (4.3)
Fixed	62 (1.9)
Host response to surgical trauma	
Fibrous adhesions	223 (6.8)
Reparative granuloma	41 (1.3)
Necrosis of long process of incus	833 (25.4)
New bony otosclerosis	175 (5.3)
Reclosure with fibrosis	38 (1.2)
Perilymphatic fistula	224 (6.8)
Faulty ossicular management	
Inadequate footplate removal	210 (6.4)
Incus luxation/subluxation	31 (0.9)
Depressed footplate into vestibule	13 (0.4)
Anatomic obstacles	
Malleus ankylosis	76 (2.3)
Incus ankylosis	11 (0.3)
Massive oval window otosclerosis	74 (2.3)
Facial nerve overhang	8 (0.2)
Round window otosclerosis	3 (0.1)
Lateralized oval window membrane	47 (1.4)
Thin ow membrane	2 (0.1)
Idiopathic	96 (2.9)

cause displacement of the prosthesis, including a problem with the distal aspect of the prosthesis (ie, fibrous tissue/new bone growth in the oval window) or the proximal (incus) side of the prosthesis (Figs. 1 and 2). Necrosis of the long process of the incus is the most common finding when the prosthesis is displaced from the incus (see Table 2).

Persistent conductive hearing loss

One of the most common causes of a persistent conductive hearing loss is an unrecognized epitympanic fixation of the malleus or incus. Other causes include incus subluxation, a loose prosthesis, a prosthesis that is too short, inadequate footplate removal, and round window otosclerosis (see Table 2). All of these conditions are amenable to revision, with the exception of round window otosclerosis. Complete obliteration of the round window niche is extremely rare, occurring in approximately 0.1% of cases (see Table 2). Both Gristwood [31] and Causse [32] have been unsuccessful in improving hearing when the round window is blocked by otosclerotic foci. Attempting to remove otosclerosis in the round window may result in deafness [32]. In general, cases with persistent conductive hearing loss after primary stapedectomy will have poorer hearing outcomes from revision, compared with cases in which there was delayed conductive hearing loss [5].

Patients with persistent conductive hearing loss after stapedectomy may also have an unrecognized superior semicircular canal dehiscence (SSCD) [33,34]. Cases have been documented of an SSCD presenting with

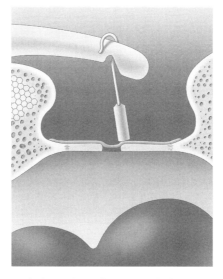

Fig. 1. Stapedectomy prosthesis displaced from oval window fenestra. (*From* Lesinski SG. Causes of conductive hearing loss after stapedectomy or stapedotomy: a prospective study of 279 consecutive surgical revisions. Otol Neurotol 2002;23:281–8; with permission.)

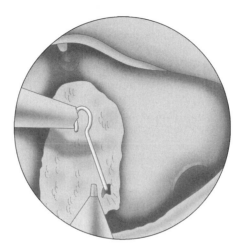

Fig. 2. Fibrotic tissue in oval window. Incus is necrosed. (*From* Lesinski SG. Causes of conductive hearing loss after stapedectomy or stapedotomy: a prospective study of 279 consecutive surgical revisions. Otol Neurotol 2002;23:281–8; with permission.)

conductive hearing loss without dizziness [34–36]. An elevation in air conduction thresholds relative to bone conduction thresholds in SSCD is believed to be caused by "shunting" of perilymph toward the superior semicircular canal (ie, a "third window") and away from the cochlea. The conductive hearing loss of SSCD may be corrected with superior semicircular canal plugging [34]. A CT scan is necessary when considering the diagnosis of SSCD (see "Radiologic evaluation" section). If an SSCD is found on CT, revision stapedectomy should not be performed.

Dizziness

Dizziness for a few days after stapedectomy is common. Poststapedectomy dizziness lasting weeks to months, however, should be considered as an indication for middle ear exploration and possible revision. Some persistent poststapedectomy dizziness may be due to fairly obvious middle ear pathology identifiable at the time of exploration. These pathologic findings may include a PLF, an overly long prosthesis, tissue reaction (eg, granuloma), or otitis media. Other conditions causing dizziness that cannot be seen during middle ear exploration include benign paroxysmal positional vertigo (BPPV), excessive aspiration of perilymph (dry labyrinth), suppurative labyrinthitis, endolymphatic hydrops (ELH), utricular or saccular adhesions, or a footplate fragment in contact with vestibular contents [37–39].

It is often difficult to determine when to consider medical therapy alone instead of surgery for cases of persistent poststapedectomy dizziness. As such, the following management guidelines are recommended. First, the presence of BPPV must be ruled out [39], because BPPV is treatable with the Epley maneuver, not middle ear exploration. If BPPV has been ruled out, then clues to the cause of dizziness may be found in the history and in audiometric findings. Typically, patients with PLF complain of a constant or intermittent feeling of disequilibrium. Auditory symptoms of a PLF may include a "tinny" quality to sound, loss of pitch, sound distortion, recruitment, and loud, roaring tinnitus [13]. The audiometric findings in cases of a PLF vary widely, from normal hearing, to conductive hearing loss, to a flat or fluctuating sensorineural hearing loss [40]. A fistula sign is often negative in patients with a PLF poststapedectomy [40]. The symptom of an overly long prosthesis is usually a vertiginous sensation during periods of increased middle ear or intracranial pressure.

When dizziness develops months to years after surgery, it is often due to a PLF [41] or, rarely, Meniere's disease. For a further discussion of vertigo after stapedectomy, please see the article elsewhere in this issue.

Sensorineural hearing loss

Possible causes of sensorineural hearing loss after stapedectomy are similar to those mentioned previously for dizziness (excluding BPPV). Middle ear exploration and revision are indicated rarely for sensorineural hearing loss, except in select situations because bone conduction thresholds are rarely, if ever, improved in these cases [16,30,42]. Improvement in speech discrimination has been reported [16], but is uncommon. The main goal of revision stapedectomy for sensorineural hearing loss is to prevent further deterioration in hearing (if hearing is still present).

Cases of anacusis without dizziness should not be explored because hearing cannot be improved. If hearing is fluctuating or progressive, then middle exploration may be considered. Fluctuating or progressive sensorineural hearing loss suggests the possibility of a potentially reversible cause, such as a PLF or an oval window granuloma. Medical treatment in the form of steroids, antibiotics, or vasodilators may be used to treat stable, mild to severe sensorineural hearing loss, with some chance for hearing improvement [43].

Distortion of sound

A patient's own voice or the sound of speech may cause a distortion or "vibration" of sound in the operated ear, an infrequent symptom after stapedectomy, but one that can be corrected with revision [4]. A short prosthesis is often a cause of this symptom and can be corrected by placing a slightly longer prosthesis. The loose-wire syndrome has been reported by McGee [44]. This syndrome may occur in patients who have a stapedectomy prosthesis that is crimped to the incus. It consists of a triad of one or more symptoms, including auditory acuity, distortion of sound, and speech discrimination, that improve temporarily with middle ear inflation [44].

Other tympanic/middle ear problems

Various other pathologies may develop after stapedectomy, such as tympanic adhesions, perforations, or cholesteatoma [45,46]. Each of these conditions can be treated with standard tympanoplasty techniques.

Contraindications for surgery

In the authors' opinion, an absolute contraindication to revision is operating on an infected or only hearing ear. The vestibule should not be opened in cases of a tympanic membrane perforation. The decision making becomes more complicated when there have been two failed revisions on the worse hearing ear. At times, the authors would recommend primary stapedectomy on the contralateral ear rather than risk a third failure because the chance of a successful hearing outcome diminishes with each revision [4–13].

Preoperative evaluation

Pertinent history and previous operative procedure

Preoperative evaluation depends on what the patient is complaining about. One important question is whether there was hearing improvement after the initial stapedectomy. Patients with the best chance for success after revision stapedectomy are those who have a conductive hearing loss that developed after an initially good hearing result.

The patient may also complain of fluctuations in hearing, or a "rattling" or distortion of sound. These symptoms may be due to a loose or short prosthesis altered by variations in middle ear pressure. When negative pressure increases, so does hearing.

PLF may also cause fluctuations in hearing. PLF most commonly causes a constant feeling of disequilibrium, worsened with head motion. A sudden drop in hearing after air travel or scuba diving is consistent with the possibility of a perilymph fistula.

When available, operative records of the previous surgery may be helpful. Some of the items to be considered when evaluating the previous operative report include

- Type and length of the prosthesis used
- Status of the footplate (floating, biscuit, obliterated requiring drill-out)
- How the footplate was managed (stapedotomy, partial or total stapedectomy)
- Use of tissue seal (which type)

All this information may be useful in determining candidacy for revision and therefore may lead to a more successful outcome. One must use caution, however, when evaluating the previous operative report because the report may be unreliable [4,47].

Physical examination

A routine examination of the ear, with special attention to the external canal, tympanic membrane, and middle ear space should be performed. An infected ear canal is a contraindication for surgery. The mobility of the malleus should be checked using a binocular microscope and air insufflation of the ear canal. Pressure fistula testing and Dix-Hallpike testing should be performed in all patients complaining of dizziness. Rinne tuning fork testing at 512 Hz and 1024 Hz is recommended to corroborate audiologic testing.

Audiologic evaluation

Air and bone pure-tone audiometry, along with word recognition testing for both ears, should be performed in all cases where revision stapedectomy is being considered. Bone conduction must be measured accurately because it is a measure of cochlear reserve. Masking must be performed properly to ensure accurate bone conduction values.

Masking is performed first by determining the amount of test signal crossover or interaural attenuation (IA). The IA is a limit to the loudness of the pure-tone/speech test signal before it will cross over to the nontest ear (NTE). It is important to remember that air-conducted signals (pure tones and speech) cross over to the opposite side by bone conduction. When IA is exceeded, masking noise is needed to prevent the NTE from hearing and responding. The IA limit depends on the type of transducer being used. When using supra-aural headphones, the IA or crossover volume limit for air-conducted pure tones is 40 dB and for air-conducted speech is 50 dB. When using insert earphones, the IA is 70 dB for air-conducted pure tones and 50 dB for speech. For bone conduction testing, the IA is zero.

The second step is to account for any present or possible ABG in the NTE, which will need to be added to the amount of test signal that is crossing over above the IA limit when masking for both air and bone conduction.

The final step is to account for the occlusion effect. When an earphone is placed in or on the NTE, an artificial improvement in the bone conduction score can occur because of the increase in the sound pressure generated by the closed external auditory canal, resulting in an increase in sound energy reaching the cochlea. The occlusion effect will occur when occluding a normal ear or one with a sensorineural loss (noting no improvement with purely conductive losses) and affects only the lower frequencies, 250 and 500 Hz.

Appropriate masking in otosclerosis is generally quite effective except in cases of a maximal ABG, either with or without a sensorineural overlay. In cases of maximal conductive involvement, it may be impossible to provide enough masking to the NTE without the masking signal crossing back over to the test ear, thereby affecting the test ear threshold. This phenomenon is termed a masking dilemma.

In addition to a complete audiometric evaluation, stapedial reflex testing should be performed on all primary cases. In the early stages of otosclerosis, various types of acoustic reflex patterns have been identified. Most recently, Lopez Gonzalez and colleagues [48] reported on and off stapedial reflexes in 18%, inverted reflexes in 46%, and absent reflexes in 27% of 188 surgically confirmed cases of otosclerosis. The "on-off" effect is a form of stapedial reflex that presents as a double positive deflection, appearing when the stimulus starts and stops, and is very frequent in the earliest stages of otospongiosis [49]. In all other stages of otosclerosis, the stapedial reflex is characteristically absent.

If reflexes are present, one should consider the possibility of an SSCD as a cause of pseudoconductive hearing loss. The dehiscence creates a "third window" in the inner ear that shunts acoustic energy through the vestibular labyrinth rather than through the cochlea. Vestibular evoked myogenic potentials (VEMP) may also be helpful in the assessment of SSCD. The VEMP threshold is typically 20 dB lower in SSCD cases than in normal subjects (70 dB versus 95 dB) [50,51].

Radiologic evaluation

A preoperative CT scan is recommended before the revision procedure, especially when the surgeon who will be performing the operation was not the previous stapes surgeon. A CT scan is useful to identify malleal fixation to the attic, incus necrosis, a long prosthesis into the vestibule, and bone formation in the oval or round windows. CT may also identify air in the vestibule, an indirect sign of PLF [52]. A CT scan with oblique views through the temporal bone can also identify the presence of an SSCD.

Histopathology of stapes procedures

The late Harold Schuknecht has shown that success in stapes surgery is improved with a thorough understanding of the histopathology of the temporal bone. Stapes surgery can be notoriously difficult, challenging even the most experienced surgeon. Mild ELH is common in stapes surgery and accounts for a drop in bone score immediately after the surgery. Evidence exists to suggest that ELH occurs routinely after stapedectomy [53]. Schuknecht and Tonndorf [54] report that inward displacement of the footplate can injure the organ of corti. Response of the host to the material implanted, such as Gelfoam, has been studied, and has demonstrated inflammatory reactions.

Nadol [55] studied the histopathology of 22 ears with either residual or recurrent conductive hearing loss after stapedectomy. The most common histopathologic correlates of conductive hearing loss after stapedectomy included resorptive osteitis of the incus at the site of prosthesis attachment (64%); obliteration of the round window by otosclerosis (23%); the presence of the prosthesis lying on a footplate fragment (23%) or abutting the bony margin of the oval window rather than centered in the fenestration (18%); and the presence of postoperative new bone formation in the oval window (14%). Round window obliteration appeared to be the cause of the largest conductive hearing loss among the different types of histopathologic correlates identified. Most of the 22 ears had multiple causes of conductive hearing loss. In general, the degree of conductive hearing loss was proportional to the number of histopathologic abnormalities identified.

Incus necrosis

Resorptive osteitis of the incus is a common finding, regardless of the prosthesis used [55]. Incus necrosis is rarely the only finding. In 13 of 14 cases of incus necrosis in Nadol's study, there was at least one other histopathologic abnormality.

Round window obliteration

The round window may be obliterated on the inner surface of the round window membrane (Nadol, personal communication, 2005), preventing the operating surgeon from visualizing the obstruction. Round window fixation on the inner surface of the membrane may account for some of the cases recorded as negative findings at the time of revision stapedectomy [14,16,25,56]. A preoperative CT before revision stapedectomy and careful intraoperative evaluation of the round window niche, including observation of a round window reflex, may be helpful in identifying round window obliteration. A negative round window reflex, however, does not necessarily predict poor hearing outcome. It is unlikely that stapes surgery will be successful in cases of complete obliteration of the cochlear canal.

Malleus fixation

Various means are available to detect malleus fixation before primary stapedectomy, although no method is infallible. Malleus fixation may be identified using air insufflation while visualizing the tympanic membrane with a binocular microscope. If a good seal is obtained, malleus fixation may be identified by the absence of movement of the manubrium with insufflation. Laser vibrometry is another more objective means to detect malleus fixation preoperatively [57].

If primary stapedectomy has been performed, malleus fixation may, at times, be identified by a postoperative ABG larger than the preoperative gap [55].

New bone formation in the oval window

New bone formation in the oval window can occur, especially in cases of a drill-out for obliterative otosclerosis in the primary procedure. The new bone is not otosclerotic, but rather, reparative new bone [38,55,58].

Benefits of laser

The authors highly recommend the use of a laser during revision stapedectomy in view of the potential for multiple pathologies at the time of revision. The laser helps to decrease bleeding, atraumatically free the
prosthesis, obliterate scar tissue around the oval window, and create the fenestration. Adhesions have been found between an oval window tissue seal
and the membranous labyrinth after stapedectomy [38]. The laser allows
atraumatic removal of the soft tissue filling the oval window, without manipulation of the adhesions extending into the inner ear. In addition, the laser may be used to sculpt the tip of an eroded incus long process. Sculpting
the incus can help with placement of the Lippy modification of the Robinson prosthesis [4]. The use of laser has been shown to improve surgical outcomes and reduce complications, compared with traditional pick or drill
techniques [4,19,21].

Revision stapedectomy surgical technique

The following is a summary of general surgical guidelines recommended
for revision stapedectomy. A more detailed discussion follows regarding
specific solutions to common problems found during revision surgery.

The authors recommend local anesthesia with intravenous (IV) sedation
for the majority of revision stapedectomy cases for two reasons. First, local/
IV sedation allows the patient to respond if dizziness develops during oval
window manipulation. Second, the surgeon may assess hearing at the time
of surgery while using local/IV sedation [59]. As in primary surgery, a tympanic flap is raised and the malleus and incus are palpated for fixation. If
abnormalities of the malleus/incus are noted, then the procedure should
proceed as described in the "Management of operative problems" section.

If the malleus and incus are intact and mobile, the laser is used to remove
adhesions or an oval window neomembrane until the margins and level of
the oval window are identified. Removal of this tissue is important because
a neomembrane may often obscure the true depths of the oval window. The
laser is also used to free the tissue surrounding the proximal end of the prosthesis. The prosthesis is then removed and the laser is used to make a fenestra
in the oval window to the level of perilymph. A stapedotomy or stapedectomy with or without tissue seal is performed, depending on the wishes of
the surgeon. A new prosthesis is placed.

If the original prosthesis is deeply imbedded in the vestibule or if there is
any dizziness on manipulation of the prosthesis, the original prosthesis
should not be removed. In these situations, the prosthesis should be de-
tached from the incus and pushed toward the promontory. A new tissue
graft is slit so that it encompasses the medial end of the original prosthesis
and is then placed over the fenestrated oval window [4]. A new prosthesis is
then placed on the tissue graft.

Management of operative problems

The following is a discussion of some specific management solutions for revision stapedectomy.

Prosthetic malfunction

Prosthetic malfunction includes any problem found with the stapes prosthesis (eg, dislodged prosthesis at the incus or oval window, short, long, or loose prosthesis). By far the most common malfunction is a dislodged prosthesis at the incus or oval window (see Table 2). Prosthesis migration out of the oval window fenestration is believed to be due to collagen contracture of the neomembrane sealing the oval window fenestration. As the neomembrane contracts, it lifts the prosthesis out of the fenestration [47]. It is believed that the thicker the tissue used to seal the oval window (fascia, fat, perichondrium, vein, in order of decreasing thickness), the more contracture and lateralization occurs [47]. However, one author has seen the opposite occurrence; in that case, the oval window neomembrane contracted medially to cover the vestibular labyrinth, causing the proximal end of the prosthesis to "float" above the neomembrane.

Treatment of prosthetic malfunction problems consists of identifying the cause of failure and treating it accordingly. A dislodged prosthesis at the incus may be due to incus necrosis, a loose crimp, or displacement out of the oval window. A loose crimp may be treated with recrimping if no other pathology is found. Displacement from the oval window is best treated with laser identification of the oval window, along with prosthesis replacement, as outlined earlier. A short or long prosthesis can be corrected by replacement with a prosthesis of proper length.

Incus necrosis

Incus erosion occurs as the incus continues to vibrate against the fixed prosthesis because of differential motion at the incus/prosthesis interface. Incus necrosis may also be the result of an inflammatory response and bone remodeling caused by a tight crimp of the prosthesis around the long process of the incus.

Different surgical techniques and prostheses are available, depending on the degree of incus necrosis. If there is minimal erosion of the incus, one solution is to apply a crimped wire higher on the incus, above the site of erosion. This practice, however, has been associated with a high rate of re-erosion [10,60,61]. Another option is placement of an incus interposition [26] or use of the Lippy modification of the Robinson bucket handle prosthesis [4,60]. This modified prosthesis has part of the well removed to allow entry of the eroded long process of the incus. Lippy and colleagues [60,62,63] have reported short-term success (70%–90% <10 dB PTA ABG) and long-term results [64] (50%–60% <10 dB PTA ABG, 3–10 years postoperatively) with the modified Lippy prosthesis for mild incus necrosis. An offset version of the Lippy modified prosthesis may be used in cases of more severe incus necrosis.

The incus can be bypassed when it is damaged severely. Incus bypass options include a malleus-to-oval window prosthesis [10] or a total ossicular reconstruction prosthesis [65]. In 1970 Feldman and Schuknecht [10] were the first to report the malleus-to-oval window technique. Two successful malleus-to-oval window prostheses include the "Smart Malleus Piston" (Gyrus-ENT, Bartlett, TN) and the titanium Clip Piston MVP (malleovestibulopexy) (Kurz Corporation, Germany). The wire end of the Smart Malleus Piston is made of nitinol, which bends upon heat contact [66]. The nitinol simplifies the crimping at the malleus.

The Clip Piston MVP is a titanium prosthesis with a clip end to attach to the manubrium, a ball joint, and a rounded shaft for placement into the oval window fenestra (Fig. 3). The clip eliminates the need for crimping and the ball joint prevents the need for bending of the prosthesis, which would compromise sound transmission. The average length of either type of malleus-to-oval window prosthesis is 6.5 mm (range 5.0 – 7.0 mm) [13,57,67].

The length of the prosthesis used for incus bypass is determined by measuring the distance between the undersurface of the manubrium and the oval window and then adding 0.5 mm to that value to account for the width of the manubrium and the stapes footplate. To place the prosthesis around the manubrium, the periosteum of the manubrium near the neck of the malleus and the overlying tympanic membrane are elevated sharply to create a space for the distal part of the prosthesis. The prosthesis is then inserted into the vestibule while positioning the distal part of the prosthesis on the manubrium. Once correctly positioned, the prosthesis is attached to the manubrium in a manner appropriate for the type of prosthesis being used. A tissue seal (eg, auricle fat) is applied around the oval window to prevent the development of a perilymph fistula.

When a total ossicular replacement prosthesis is used to bypass the incus, a tissue graft must be used over the stapes fenestra. The tissue seal prevents subluxation into the vestibule. The head of the total ossicular replacement prosthesis can be placed under the tympanic membrane exclusively, or a portion of the prosthesis head can be stabilized under the manubrium (preferable). Battaglia and colleagues [65] recommend packing the eustachian tube with moistened, pressed Gelfoam. The Gelfoam is used to provide middle ear stasis during the postoperative period, to prevent displacement of the prosthesis secondary to transmitted pressure changes. In general, the hearing results using the malleus-to-oval window and total ossicular replacement prosthesis are similar [68].

One final solution for incus necrosis is the use of bone cement to reconstruct the long process of the incus. Both hydroxyapatite cement [69] (Mimix; Walter Lorenz Surgical; Jacksonville, FL) and glass ionomeric cement [70,71] (OtoCem, Oto-Tech, Raleigh, NC) have been used to reconstruct the incus

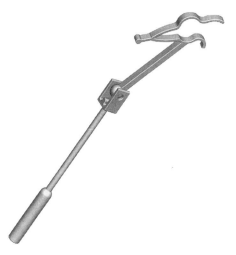

Fig. 3. The titanium Clip Piston MVP. (Kurz Corporation, Germany) for malleus-to-oval window replacement. The distal end consists of a Clip mechanism that allows a crimp-free connection to the malleus handle. The middle section is a ball joint, which eliminates the need to bend the implant. (Courtesy of Kurz Corporation, Germany; with permission.)

long process. The most successful outcomes occur when a crimp-on prosthesis is placed on the incus remnant and stabilized with the cement, rather than placing the prosthesis on the cement itself [69,71].

Malleus/incus fixation

Malleus or incus fixation may go unrecognized at the time of the initial operation, or the fixation may develop as a result of trauma from the primary surgery [28]. The fixation in previously operated ears occurs in congenitally susceptible ears as a result of surgical manipulation or bleeding [28].

Malleus fixation may be detected preoperatively through air insufflation of the ear canal, or more precisely, with the use of laser Doppler vibrometry [57]. The displacement amplitude of the partially or totally fixed manubrium is significantly lower at middle frequencies with laser Doppler vibrometry than in normal subjects or in patients with otosclerotic stapes fixation [57].

When partial or total malleus fixation is suspected or identified, the authors recommend the endaural approach, a superior tympanostomy flap (3 o'clock to 9 o'clock positions), and a superior canaloplasty, as advocated by Fisch and colleagues [57]. Malleus fixation occurs most often because of calcification of the anterior malleal ligament. Incus fixation/subluxation can often be identified only after the incudomalleal joint is visualized properly. The endaural/superior canaloplasty approach offers the advantage of direct visual control of the mobility of the anterior malleal process, the anterior malleal ligament, and the incudomalleal joint. If there is any doubt about the mobility of the malleus or incus, the incudo-prosthetic joint should be separated.

Treatment of malleus/incus fixation or incus subluxation consists of either placement of a malleus-to-oval window prosthesis or a total ossicular prosthesis, thereby bypassing the lateral ossicular chain. If a malleus-to-oval window prosthesis is to be used, the malleus fixation must be corrected by removal of the malleus head, anterior malleal process, and ligament [57]. The anterior malleal process and ligament must be removed to ensure mobility of the manubrium [57].

Obliterative otosclerosis/massive bony regrowth

Obliterative otosclerosis or massive bony regrowth is found commonly at the time of revision if the primary case was that of obliterative otosclerosis (Fig. 4) [25]. Some investigators recommend avoiding drilling the oval window at the time of revision stapedectomy [14,25,29]. Other investigators, however, report successful hearing results when a drill-out of obliterative otosclerosis is performed for revision stapedectomy [6,10,18,27,72]. Wide saucerization of the oval window during a drill-out should be avoided because of the higher incidence of immediate or delayed sensorineural hearing loss. A small fenestra should be made, preferably in the posteroinferior portion of the footplate to avoid the membranous labyrinth. The last remaining portion of bone should be removed with a laser to minimize labyrinth trauma.

Suspected perilymphatic fistula

PLF is the most common cause of persistent (lasting 4 or more weeks) or delayed dizziness [41] after stapedectomy. An identifiable PLF has been

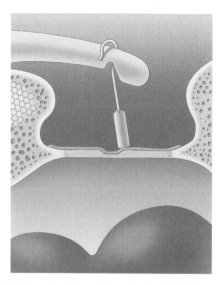

Fig. 4. Bony regrowth in the oval window. (*From* Lesinski SG. Causes of conductive hearing loss after stapedectomy or stapedotomy: a prospective study of 279 consecutive surgical revisions. Otol Neurotol 2002;23:281–8; with permission.)

reported in 6.8% of revision stapes surgery cases (see Table 2). Because there are no diagnostic tests for PLF, the suspicion of a PLF rests on the symptoms outlined earlier in the "Dizziness" section.

When revision surgery is performed for poststapedectomy dizziness, the oval window must be explored carefully. The application of a slight pressure over the long process of the incus may help to reveal a PLF. If a PLF is found, the oval window niche should be covered with a tissue seal followed by fibrin glue. If no PLF is identified, fibrin glue should be used to seal the oval window region because a microfistula may be present [40]. Often, dizziness will improve if these techniques are used [40].

Special situations

Multiple revisions

In general, the likelihood of a successful hearing outcome diminishes with each revision [4–13]. The authors, therefore, rarely recommend a third revision if there have been two previous failures.

Presumed sympathetic cochleovestibulitis after multiple revision stapedectomies has been reported [73]. Sympathetic cochleovestibulitis is thought to develop from an activation of the humoral or cell-mediated immune response to inner ear antigens exposed as a result of surgery [74,75]. One group of investigators has theorized that exposure of inner ear antigens to the systemic immune system at the time of stapedectomy may result in an autoimmune-mediated hearing loss in both the operated and contralateral ear of predisposed individuals [73].

The elderly patient

Data for elderly patients undergoing a revision stapedectomy are very sparse. Lippy and colleagues [76] recently evaluated hearing results for 120 elderly subjects (age greater than 70) who had a revision stapedectomy. The authors report a mean 3-frequency PTA improvement of 17 dB. The average postoperative ABG was 6.5 dB. Seventy-one percent of their subjects had an ABG of less than 10 dB, and 90% had an ABG of less than 20 dB. They were able to evaluate 69 of these subjects for a long period of time (mean 6.7 years). The PTA decreased approximately 1 dB per year, which is similar to studies of younger subjects. The results indicate that revision stapedectomy in the elderly is usually successful.

Summary

Revision stapedectomy can be a technically demanding operation. The surgeon must be prepared for numerous pathologic conditions. Appropriate preoperative patient counseling is a must. The best chance for hearing improvement is in those cases that have a delayed conductive hearing loss after primary stapedectomy. The authors would seldom advise revision for profound sensorineural hearing or in cases of two previous revisions.

References

[1] Shea JJ. Fenestration of the oval window. Ann Otol Rhinol Laryngol 1958;67:932–5.
[2] Meyer TA, Lambert PR. Primary and revision stapedectomy in elderly patients. Curr Opin Otolaryngol Head Neck Surg 2004;12:387–92.
[3] Equilibrium AAoOHaNSCoHa. Committee on Hearing and Equilibrium guidelines for the evaluation of results of treatment of conductive hearing loss. Otolaryngol Head Neck Surg 1995;113:186–7.
[4] Lippy WH, Battista RA, Berenholz L, et al. Twenty-year review of revision stapedectomy. Otol Neurotol 2003;24:560–6.
[5] Han WW, Incesulu A, McKenna MJ, et al. Revision stapedectomy: intraoperative findings, results, and review of the literature. Laryngoscope 1997;107:1185–92.
[6] Glasscock ME 3rd, McKennan KX, Levine SC. Revision stapedectomy surgery. Otolaryngol Head Neck Surg 1987;96:141–8.
[7] Sheehy JL, Nelson RA, House HP. Revision stapedectomy: a review of 258 cases. Laryngoscope 1981;91:43–51.
[8] Crabtree JA, Britton BH, Powers WH. An evaluation of revision stapes surgery. Laryngoscope 1980;90:224–7.
[9] Lesinski SG, Stein JA. Stapedectomy revision with the CO2 laser. Laryngoscope 1989;99: 13–9.
[10] Feldman BA, Schuknecht HF. Experiences with revision stapedectomy procedures. Laryngoscope 1970;80:1281–91.
[11] Somers T, Govaerts P, de Varebeke SJ, et al. Revision stapes surgery. J Laryngol Otol 1997; 111:233–9.
[12] Pedersen CB. Revision surgery in otosclerosis–operative findings in 186 patients. Clin Otolaryngol Allied Sci 1994;19:446–50.
[13] Farrior J, Sutherland A. Revision stapes surgery. Laryngoscope 1991;101:1155–61.
[14] Bhardwaj BK, Kacker SK. Revision stapes surgery. J Laryngol Otol 1988;102:20–4.
[15] Cokkeser Y, Naguib M, Aristegui M, et al. Revision stapes surgery: a critical evaluation. Otolaryngol Head Neck Surg 1994;111:473–7.
[16] Dawes JD, Curry AR. Types of stapedectomy failure and prognosis of revision operations. J Laryngol Otol 1974;88:213–26.
[17] De La Cruz A, Fayad JN. Revision stapedectomy. Otolaryngol Head Neck Surg 2000;123: 728–32.
[18] Derlacki EL. Revision stapes surgery: problems with some solutions. Laryngoscope 1985;95: 1047–53.
[19] Haberkamp TJ, Harvey SA, Khafagy Y. Revision stapedectomy with and without the CO2 laser: an analysis of results. Am J Otol 1996;17:225–9.
[20] Hammerschlag PE, Fishman A, Scheer AA. A review of 308 cases of revision stapedectomy. Laryngoscope 1998;108:1794–800.
[21] Horn KL, Gherini SG, Franz DC. Argon laser revision stapedectomy. Am J Otol 1994;15: 383–8.
[22] Hough JV, Dyer RK Jr. Stapedectomy. Causes of failure and revision surgery in otosclerosis. Otolaryngol Clin North Am 1993;26:453–70.
[23] Langman AW, Lindeman RC. Revision stapedectomy. Laryngoscope 1993;103:954–8.
[24] Lesinski SG. Revision stapedectomy. Curr Opin Otolaryngol Head Neck Surg 2003;11: 347–54.
[25] Lippy WH, Schuring AG, Ziv M. Stapedectomy Revision. Am J Otol 1980;2:15–21.

[26] Palva T, Ramsay H. Revision surgery for otosclerosis. Acta Otolaryngol 1990;110:416–20.

[27] Prasad S, Kamerer DB. Results of revision stapedectomy for conductive hearing loss. Otolaryngol Head Neck Surg 1993;109:742–7.

[28] Shea JJ Jr. The management of repeat stapes operations. Laryngoscope 1968;78:808–12.

[29] Vartiainen E, Nuutinen J, Virtaniemi J. Long-term results of revision stapes surgery. J Laryngol Otol 1992;106:971–3.

[30] Lippy WH, Schuring AG. Stapedectomy revision following sensorineural hearing loss. Otolaryngol Head Neck Surg 1984;92:580–2.

[31] Gristwood RE. Otosclerosis (otospongiosis): general considerations. In: Alberti PW, Ruben R, editors. Otologic medicine and surgery. New York: Churchill Livingstone; 1988. p. 30–44.

[32] Causse JB, Causse JR, Wiet R. Special conditions in otosclerosis surgery. In: Wiet RJ, Causse JB, Shambaugh G, et al, editors. Otosclerosis (otospongiosis). Alexandria, VA: American Academy of Otolaryngology-Head and Neck Surgery Foundation, Inc.; 1991. p. 20–5.

[33] Halmagyi GM, Aw ST, McGarvie LA, et al. Superior semicircular canal dehiscence simulating otosclerosis. J Laryngol Otol 2003;117:553–7.

[34] Mikulec AA, McKenna MJ, Ramsey MJ, et al. Superior semicircular canal dehiscence presenting as conductive hearing loss without vertigo. Otol Neurotol 2004;25:121–9.

[35] Rosowski JJ, Songer JE, Nakajima HH, et al. Clinical, experimental, and theoretical investigations of the effect of superior semicircular canal dehiscence on hearing mechanisms. Otol Neurotol 2004;25:323–32.

[36] Minor LB, Carey JP, Cremer PD, et al. Dehiscence of bone overlying the superior canal as a cause of apparent conductive hearing loss. Otol Neurotol 2003;24:270–8.

[37] Belal A, Ylikoski J. Post stapedectomy dizziness: A histopathologic report. Am J Otol 1982;3: 1987–191.

[38] Linthicum FH Jr. Histologic evidence of the cause of failure in stapes surgery. Ann Otol Rhinol Laryngol 1971;80:67–77.

[39] Atacan E, Sennaroglu L, Genc A, et al. Benign paroxysmal positional vertigo after stapedectomy. Laryngoscope 2001;111:1257–9.

[40] Albera R, Canale A, Lacilla M, et al. Delayed vertigo after stapes surgery. Laryngoscope 2004;114:860–2.

[41] Roulleau P, Martin CH. In: Arnette, editor. L'otospongiose Otosclérose. Paris, 1994.

[42] Schuknecht HF. Sensorineural hearing loss following stapedectomy. Acta Otolaryngol 1962; 54:336–48.

[43] Mann WJ, Amedee RG, Fuerst G, et al. Hearing loss as a complication of stapes surgery. Otolaryngol Head Neck Surg 1996;115:324–8.

[44] McGee TM. The loose wire syndrome. Laryngoscope 1981;91:1478–83.

[45] von Haacke NP, Wilson JA, Murray JA, et al. Cholesteatoma following stapedectomy. J Laryngol Otol 1987;101:708–10.

[46] Ferguson BJ, Gillespie CA, Kenan PD, et al. Mechanisms of cholesteatoma formation following stapedectomy. Am J Otol 1986;7:420–4.

[47] Lesinski SG. Causes of conductive hearing loss after stapedectomy or stapedotomy: a prospective study of 279 consecutive surgical revisions. Otol Neurotol 2002;23:281–8.

[48] Lopez Gonzalez MA, Garcia Lopez MC, Rodriguez Munoz ML. Evaluation of the morphology of stapedial reflex in otosclerosis. Provoked otosclerotic stapedial reflex. Acta Otorrinolaringol Esp 2002;53:5–10.

[49] Camicas M. Acoustic and mechanical interpretation of the "on-off" effect. Rev Laryngol Otol Rhinol (Bord) 1992;113:355–8.

[50] Ostrowski VB, Byskosh A, Hain TC. Tullio phenomenon with dehiscence of the superior semicircular canal. Otol Neurotol 2001;22:61.

[51] Brantberg K, Bergenius J, Tribukait A. Vestibular-evoked myogenic potentials in patients with dehiscence of the superior semicircular canal. Acta Otolaryngol 1999;119:633.

[52] Kosling S, Woldag K, Meister EF, et al. Tile value of computed tomography in patients with persistent vertigo after stapes surgery. Invest Radiol 1995;30:712–5.

[53] Hohmann A. Inner ear reactions to stapes surgery. In: Schuknecht HF, editor. Otosclerosis. Boston: Little, Brown; 1962. p. 305–17.

[54] Schuknecht HF, Tonndorf J. An experimental and clinical study of deafness from lesions of the cochlear nerve. J Laryngol Otol 1960;69:75–9.

[55] Nadol JB Jr. Histopathology of residual and recurrent conductive hearing loss after stapedectomy. Otol Neurotol 2001;22:162–9.

[56] Pearman K, Dawes JD. Post-stapedectomy conductive deafness and results of revision surgery. J Laryngol Otol 1982;96:405–10.

[57] Fisch U, Acar GO, Huber AM. Malleostapedotomy in revision surgery for otosclerosis. Otol Neurotol 2001;22:776–85.

[58] Lindsay JR. Histopathologic findings following stapedectomy and polyethylene tube inserts in the human. Ann Otol Rhinol Laryngol 1961;70:785–807.

[59] Lippy WH, Schuring AG, Rizer FM. Intraoperative audiometry. Laryngoscope 1995;105: 214–6.

[60] Lippy WH, Schuring AG. Prosthesis for the problem incus in stapedectomy. Arch Otolaryngol 1974;100:237–9.

[61] Harrison WH. Prosthesis versus patient's tissue in ossicular reconstruction. Laryngoscope 1969;79:60–84.

[62] Lippy WH, Schuring AG. Solving ossicular problems in stapedectomy. Laryngoscope 1983; 93:1147–50.

[63] Lippy WL, Schuring AG. Stapedectomy revision of the wire-Gelfoam prosthesis. Otolaryngol Head Neck Surg 1983;91:9–13.

[64] Krieger LW, Lippy WH, Schuring AG, et al. Revision stapedectomy for incus erosion: long-term hearing. Otolaryngol Head Neck Surg 1998;119:370–3.

[65] Battaglia A, McGrew BM, Jackson CG. Reconstruction of the entire ossicular conduction mechanism. Laryngoscope 2003;113:654–8.

[66] Knox GW, Reitan H. Shape-memory stapes prosthesis for otosclerosis surgery. Laryngoscope 2005;115:1340–6.

[67] Kohan D, Sorin A. Revision stapes surgery: the malleus to oval window wire-piston technique. Laryngoscope 2003;113:1520–4.

[68] Sheehy JL. Stapedectomy: incus bypass procedures. a report of 203 operations. Laryngoscope 1982;92:258–62.

[69] Goebel JA, Jacob A. Use of Mimix hydroxyapatite bone cement for difficult ossicular reconstruction. Otolaryngol Head Neck Surg 2005;132:727–34.

[70] Feghali JG, Barrs DM, Beatty CW, et al. Bone cement reconstruction of the ossicular chain: a preliminary report. Laryngoscope 1998;108:829–36.

[71] Chen DA, Arriaga MA. Technical refinements and precautions during ionomeric cement reconstruction of incus erosion during revision stapedectomy. Laryngoscope 2003;113:848–52.

[72] Pedersen CB. Revision surgery in otosclerosis–an investigation of the factors which influence the hearing result. Clin Otolaryngol Allied Sci 1996;21:385–8.

[73] Richards ML, Moorhead JE, Antonelli PJ. Sympathetic cochleolabyrinthitis in revision stapedectomy surgery. Otolaryngol Head Neck Surg 2002;126:273–80.

[74] Schindler JS, Niparko JK. Transverse temporal bone fractures (left) with subsequent progressive SNHL, consistent with sympathetic cochleolabyrinthitis. Arch Otolaryngol 1998; 124:816–8.

[75] Harris JP, Low NC, House WF. Contralateral hearing loss following inner ear injury: sympathetic cochleolabyrinthitis? Am J Otol 1985;6:371–7.

[76] Lippy WH, Wingate J, Burkey JM, et al. Stapedectomy revision in elderly patients. Laryngoscope 2002;112:1100–3.

[77] Lesinski SG, Palmer A. CO2 laser for otosclerosis: safe energy parameters. Laryngoscope 1989;99:9–12.

[78] McGee TM, Diaz-Ordaz EA, Kartush JM. The role of KTP laser in revision stapedectomy. Otolaryngol Head Neck Surg 1993;109:839–43.

[79] Silverstein H, Bendet E, Rosenberg S, et al. Revision stapes surgery with and without laser: a comparison. Laryngoscope 1994;104:1431–8.

[80] Glasscock ME 3rd, Storper IS, Haynes DS, et al. Twenty-five years of experience with stapedectomy. Laryngoscope 1995;105:899–904.

[81] Wiet RJ, Kubek DC, Lemberg P, et al. A meta-analysis review of revision stapes surgery with argon laser: effectiveness and safety. Am J Otol 1997;18:166–71.

[82] Magliulo G, Cristofari P, Terranova G. Functional hearing results in revision stapes surgery. Am J Otol 1997;18:408–12.

[83] Nissen RL. Argon laser in difficult stapedotomy cases. Laryngoscope 1998;108:1669–73.

[84] Shah N. Revision stapedectomy for late conductive deafness. J Laryngol Otol 1974;88:207–12.

[85] Birt BD, Smitheringale A. Stapedectomy - a 10 year review at Sunnybrook Hospital. J Otolaryngol 1980;9:387–94.

[86] Rauch SD, Bartley ML. Argon laser stapedectomy: comparison to traditional fenestration techniques. Am J Otol 1992;13:556–60.

ELSEVIER
SAUNDERS

Otolaryngol Clin N Am
39 (2006) 699–712

OTOLARYNGOLOGIC
CLINICS
OF NORTH AMERICA

Revision Ossiculoplasty

Ravi N. Samy, MD, FACS*,
Myles L. Pensak, MD, FACS

*The Neuroscience Institute, Department of Otolaryngology,
University of Cincinnati/Cincinnati Children's Hospital Medical Center,
Cincinnati, OH, USA*

Although ossiculoplasty was attempted initially in the early 1900s, it was not until the era of Wullstein [1] and Zollner [2] in the 1950s that it became commonplace and relatively well understood. Since then, there have been numerous technologic advances and a gain in the understanding of ossiculoplasty, also known as ossicular chain reconstruction (OCR). However, even in primary cases performed by an experienced otologic surgeon, successful OCR with resulting long-term stability can be a daunting task. This is even more true for the occasional otologic surgeon and for revision cases. Typically, the most common condition requiring revision OCR is chronic suppurative otitis media (COM) with or without cholesteatoma. Primary and revision OCR is performed also for blunt and penetrating trauma-induced conductive hearing loss (CHL), congenital defects (eg, atresia), and benign and malignant tumors. Typically, reconstruction in ears with COM is more difficult than in ears without infection.

The anatomic goal of OCR is to restore the middle ear transformer mechanism. OCR is not performed if cochlear function is poor, particularly with regards to word discrimination. OCR is also contraindicated in an only hearing ear; a hearing aid is the preferred option in this instance. Patients with bilateral CHL should have the worse hearing ear operated on first; an alternative to this approach is to operate on the more diseased ear in patients with bilateral COM [3].

The goal of revision OCR is the same as for primary OCR: to obtain both objective (audiologic, clinical examination) and subjective success. Although some surgeons avoid revision OCR in the pediatric population because of concerns about the aggressive recurrence of chronic ear disease (particularly in those under the age of 5 years), others perform OCR to minimize the

---

* Corresponding author.
E-mail address: ravinsamy@mac.com (R.N. Samy).

doi:10.1016/j.otc.2006.05.005
oto.theclinics.com

potential for deficits in acquiring language and to improve speech production and school performance.

Several issues must be considered before proceeding with revision OCR:

- Realistic expectations for the patient and surgeon, including chance for failure
- Eradication of chronic ear disease or cholesteatoma
- Possibility of staging to maximize chances of success
- Discussion of alternative methods of sound amplification (ie, hearing aids, including bone-anchored hearing aid (BAHA) placement)

The only surgically attainable goal may be control of infection, particularly in revision procedures involving COM. In some patients, amplification may be indicated, instead of an attempt at revision OCR [3]. To maximize the chances of success of revision OCR, the surgeon must understand the factor or factors that may have contributed to failure of the initial OCR, including persistent or recurrent COM, excessive fibrosis, eustachian tube dysfunction (ETD), and poor surgical technique [4]. The surgeon must also consider each of the following anatomic factors as potential contributors to OCR failure, singly or in combination: middle ear, mastoid, tympanic membrane (TM), remnant ossicular chain, and type of prosthesis. However, success correlates more often to middle ear or mastoid pathology and aeration than to the prosthesis itself [5].

Preoperative evaluation and prognosis assessment

A thorough preoperative history is performed first. Comorbidities (eg, diabetes, coronary artery disease, and so forth) must be considered. The benefits of surgery must outweigh the risks of surgery and anesthesia. Preoperative clearance by a primary care physician, specialist (eg, cardiologist), and anesthesiologist may be warranted. Patients are advised against smoking, to prevent postoperative wound healing complications and to eradicate the negative effect smoking has on eustachian tube function and middle ear disease [6]. All available outside records, including the prior operative report, should be reviewed. A detailed head and neck physical examination, with emphasis on the otologic portion, is performed. Otomicroscopic evaluation with pneumatic otoscopy and tuning fork tests is conducted. Detailed audiologic testing with pure-tone air and bone conduction, tympanometry, speech recognition, and word recognition is performed. In revision cases, CT scanning (in the axial and coronal planes, 0.5 mm or 1 mm cuts, and bone windows) is performed. The scan can assist in determining areas of tegmen erosion, facial nerve dehiscence, otic capsule erosion, and prosthesis position. MRI with gadolinium can be ordered if there is concern about encephalocele formation or impending intracranial complications.

The chances of surgical success are related to the severity of pre-existing chronic ear disease, ETD, and other complicating factors. Stratification systems have been developed for prognosis and to compare results among patients, surgeons, and prostheses. Classification systems developed for prognostic purposes are used variably, and include factors such as middle ear disease (granulation tissue, effusion, otorrhea), smoking, presence of a perforation, cholesteatoma, ossicular defects, and previous surgery. The greater the number of adverse factors, the less the chance of a good post-operative hearing result. These patients may do much better with a hearing aid. The goal of a classification system is to improve preoperative assessment and prognostication for an individual patient, and to allow better comparisons among different prostheses, surgeons, and for research and reporting purposes. One such method of assessment was reported by Black [7] in 1992, who reviewed 535 ossiculoplasties. He identified 12 features and divided them into five groups: S-surgical, P-prosthetic, I-infection, T-tissue, E-Eustachian tube (SPITE). He compared the results for his patients implanted with plastipore prostheses with the results for those implanted with hydroxylapatite (HA) prostheses; he found no significant difference between the two groups, when accounting for the different factors.

Eustachian tube

A properly functioning eustachian tube is the most important factor in the creation and maintenance of aeration in the middle ear space. Without adequate eustachian tube function, one cannot obtain a long-term improvement in hearing results with revision OCR. Adequate eustachian tube function ultimately will determine the size of the middle ear space. The minimal amount of air required in the middle ear space for OCR is approximately 0.4 mL. The type of surgical approach used also affects middle ear volume (and the size of the prosthesis needed). For example, canal wall down techniques narrow the middle ear space.

ETD contributes to OCR failure by narrowing the middle ear space and contributing to prosthesis extrusion. Methods to treat and improve ETD include treatment of allergies, laryngopharyngeal reflux, smoking, and obstruction of the middle ear and nasopharyngeal orifices (eg, due to granulation tissue/hypertrophic mucosa and adenoid hypertrophy, respectively). Direct medical or surgical treatment of the eustachian tube to improve function has been proposed (eg, tuboplasty); however, it remains to be seen whether these options will adequately treat this elusive problem for the long term. Another option to alleviate ETD is to place a ventilation tube at the time of OCR or postoperatively, if needed. Some surgeons tend to avoid placement of ventilation tubes because of the possibility of increased risk of otorrhea and the need for water precautions.

Although ETD plays the most important role in chronic ear disease and affects OCR results, no manner exists in which to quantify eustachian tube function objectively. Evaluation of contralateral ear function, assessment of TM position and mobility, the existence of retraction pockets, the ability of the patient to insufflate the middle ear (Valsalva maneuver), or forced movement of air through the eustachian tube (politzerization) can all be used in the assessment.

Middle ear and mastoid disease

Another key factor in successful revision OCR is the appropriate treatment of middle ear and mastoid ear disease, such as hypertrophic mucosa, granulation tissue, debris, tympanosclerosis, adhesions, fibrosis, and cholesteatoma. Surgical eradication of the pathologic processes may reduce the risk of recurrence by removing biofilm formation, including that formed by Pseudomonas. In chronic ear disease, eradication of disease takes precedence over reconstruction of the hearing mechanism. Residual or recurrent ear pathology can cause failure of prosthesis placement by causing prosthesis extrusion, displacing the TM, or eroding the remnant ossicular chain. Active COM can cause a resorptive osteitis of the ossicles [3].

Tympanic membrane

The TM can contribute to OCR failure through lateralization or retraction. TM perforations also contribute to failure. TM perforation that occurs secondary to the prosthesis is probably caused by pressure necrosis and not a reaction to the prosthesis itself [8]. Some surgeons use cartilage to minimize TM-related complications (Fig. 1). Cartilage can be used in reconstruction to minimize medialization of the TM (by increasing the stiffness of the TM), reduce the incidence of prosthesis extrusion, and minimize the chance of recurrent retraction pocket formation and the subsequent creation of cholesteatoma. Martin and colleagues [9] reported on 180 subjects who underwent TM reconstruction with cartilage, fascia, or perichondrium. After

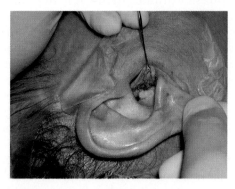

Fig. 1. Incision made over conchal cartilage to harvest cartilage for placement on head of prosthesis. Tragal cartilage is more commonly used. Care is taken to avoid using lateral third of tragal cartilage, which can cause postoperative cosmetic changes.

3 years of follow-up, the investigators reported at least a 33% decrease in retraction pocket formation in subjects undergoing TM reconstruction with cartilage. Some prostheses (eg, titanium) require the placement of cartilage, whereas others do not (eg, HA). If cartilage is used to reduce prosthesis extrusion and not to reconstruct the entire TM, the cartilage can be smaller in diameter; it needs to be large enough to cover the head of the prosthesis only. Cartilage is placed between the prosthesis and TM, after the prosthesis is positioned. Criticisms of cartilage use include a decreased ability to visualize the prosthesis during its placement (making the procedure more difficult); reduced ability to place a ventilation tube postoperatively; and hindered visualization of the middle ear space and of recurrent cholesteatoma in the postoperative period.

With TM perforations, especially large perforations, the malleus is medialized by unopposed action of the tensor tympani muscle; this narrows the middle ear space. To place the malleus in a more lateral position and increase the size of the prosthesis used, the surgeon can lyse the tensor tympani tendon or resect a portion of the manubrium.

Remnant ossicular chain

The more normal, intact, and mobile the remnant ossicular chain, the better one's chance at hearing restoration. Ossicular abnormalities can exist as discontinuity or fixation. Ossicular defects can occur singularly or in combination. When performing a revision OCR, the entire remnant ossicular chain must be palpated to assess for mobility and use in the reconstruction. Discontinuity occurs most commonly because of (1) an eroded incudostapedial (IS) joint (approximately 80% of cases), (2) absent incus (lenticular process > long process > body), (3) absent incus and stapes superstructure, or (4) absent malleus.

Ossicular fixation can be caused by adhesions (particularly in the epitympanum), calcifications (tympanosclerosis), abnormal ossicular formation (eg, atretic ears), or bone dust from prior surgical procedures, with resultant osteoneogenesis [3]. If the malleus is fixed, the attic is inspected. If the malleus head cannot be mobilized by freeing it from its attachments, the head can be resected (at the neck). The tensor tympani tendon can also be lysed if needed. Isolated fixation of the malleus can cause a CHL of up to 25 dB [3]. If incus fixation is noted intraoperatively, the IS joint is divided first, to prevent transmission of energy to the vestibule, which can cause iatrogenic sensorineural hearing loss and tinnitus. It is best to remove and replace the incus if incus mobility cannot be improved.

If the stapes is fixed because of otosclerosis or tympanosclerosis, stapes surgery (mobilization, stapedotomy, or stapedectomy) will need to be performed. Stapes fixation can result in CHL of up to 50 dB. No removal of footplate should ever be performed in the presence of an active ear infection (including a dry TM perforation) because of the risk of labyrinthitis and subsequent profound hearing loss. These patients will need staging of their ear surgery. If the footplate is removed, perichondrium or cartilage is used because of their greater rigidity compared with vein graft or temporalis fascia (preventing prosthesis displacement into the vestibule) [5]. This procedure is more challenging and is performed rarely, compared with other types of ossiculoplasties. Prosthesis length is determined before removing the footplate to minimize the amount of time the vestibule is open.

Prostheses

Ideally, implants should be biocompatible, inert, inexpensive, and easy to handle and use; they should resist adhesion formation, resorption, or fixation; and they should allow for tissue ingrowth, and stabilization and long-term hearing improvement [8]. No single implant meets all the above criteria. The numerous types of prostheses, in terms of both design and construction, attest to this problem. No evidence exists that one type of prosthesis performs significantly better than another in the long term [10]; each prosthesis type has its advantages and disadvantages. Stiffness, mass, tension, position, and coupling (among TM, prosthesis, and remnant ossicular chain) all affect the hearing result [3]. Different prostheses are used, based on the variable ossicular defects. Usually, the more minimal the ossicular defect, the better the long-term hearing results.

The Appelbaum HA prosthesis, introduced in 1993, is used to reconstruct the IS joint and the lever mechanism (instead of using an incus interposition graft) [3]. It is available in two sizes and connects the remnant incus long process to the stapes head. It has also been used successfully in pediatric cases with an average air-bone gap of 15dB at 2.5 years of follow-up [11]. The Kurz angular prosthesis (Germany), made of gold and titanium, can also be used to reconstruct the IS joint (Fig. 2).

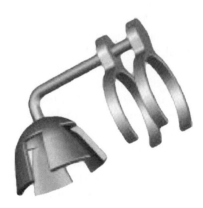

Fig. 2. Kurz angular prosthesis. (Courtesy of Kurz Medical, Inc., Norcross, GA; with permission.)

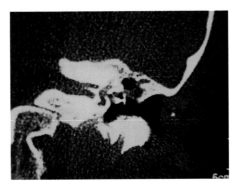

Fig. 3. Left coronal, nonenhanced CT scan of a pediatric patient with displaced partial ossicular reconstruction prosthesis and recurrence of cholesteatoma. The patient has undergone revision tympanomastoidectomy and will have prosthesis replacement at her third-stage procedure.

If there is too much erosion of the long process, the incus needs to be removed and a partial ossicular reconstruction prosthesis placed between the TM or malleus and the stapes capitulum (Fig. 3). A total ossicular reconstruction prosthesis is used for ears with both the incus and stapes superstructure missing (Fig. 4). The total ossicular reconstruction prosthesis is coupled between the malleus or TM and the stapes footplate. Patients who require placement of a total ossicular reconstruction prosthesis have, on average, the worst hearing result after reconstruction.

Sizing the prosthesis is a learned skill, and its importance should not be underestimated; inappropriate sizing can cause failure in hearing improvement. Although some surgeons measure the actual distance between the remnant ossicle and the TM, others trim the prosthesis, assess for proper

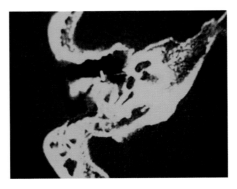

Fig. 4. Nonenhanced axial CT scan of a right ear in a patient who noted only short-term improvement in hearing after placement of a total ossicular reconstruction prosthesis. Note the malposition of the prosthesis shaft in relation to the footplate.

fit, and then trim additional material as necessary. The proper prosthesis length is such that the TM is slightly tented after prosthesis placement. A key amount of tension is needed. Gelfoam packing can be used for support. If the prosthesis is too short, the hearing result will be poor, because the remnant ossicular chain and the TM will not be coupled. If the prosthesis is too long, footplate erosion, stapes avulsion (with subsequent risk of sensorineural hearing loss) or extrusion of the prosthesis through the TM may occur.

The two main categories of prosthetic materials are: (1) biologic (autografts and homografts) and (2) synthetic (alloplasts or allografts). Autograft materials include cortical bone chips, native ossicles (usually the incus), and cartilage (from tragus or concha) [12,13]. Although resorption of autograft materials can occur, particularly with cartilage, the material is biocompatible, readily available, low in cost, and has a low risk of extrusion [3,13,14]. Autografts have shown good success. In 45 subjects, Romanet and associates [13] reported a 2-year success rate (defined as an air-bone gap of 20 dB or less) of 89%, with no cases of extrusion. However, modifying an ossicle for use can be challenging and involves the use of a drill for prosthesis modification, with risk of thermal injury and resultant resorption [3]. Many surgeons limit their use of autografts because of concerns about residual cholesteatoma on the ossicles as well as the time and expense in obtaining and sculpting the material. Surgeon, anesthesia, and operating room time are all used during fashioning of an autograft for use.

The other biologic materials, homograft ossicles and cartilage, were first used in the 1960s. They are not as popular in the US as they once were because of concerns about HIV transmission and prion spread (and subsequent Creutzfeldt-Jakob disease). However, some surgeons state that autoclaving or treating the homografts with formaldehyde should eradicate viruses, prions, and residual cholesteatoma [15]. Homografts are typically available as cadaveric TM and ossicles, cartilage, and cortical bone. They can be obtained presculpted or modified intraoperatively. Although they have many of the same advantages and disadvantages as autografts, they arguably have a higher resorption rate. Chiossone [16] reviewed 411 ossiculoplasties with homograft ossicles. Sixty-eight percent of the subjects had a follow-up after more than 5 years and of these, 88% had prostheses still in place. (The remaining patients had prostheses that were removed because of disease, necrosis, or extrusion.)

Alloplastic materials have been used since 1952 for OCR [5]. Typically, studies have shown no significant differences among synthetic prostheses in extrusion risk, failure rates, and short- and long-term hearing results, when comparing ears similar in ossicular defects and disease. In the presence of ear disease (ie, COM), these prostheses do not function as well in OCR as when used for nondiseased ears. Compared with autografts or homografts, synthetic prostheses have a higher incidence of extrusion [3]. Prostheses are made of numerous artificial substances, including Teflon, polyethylene, metal wire, polycel, carbon, bioactive glass, Ceravital, and aluminum oxide ceramic [8]. Most current prostheses are made of titanium, plastipore, and HA (singly or in combination), with dense HA the most commonly used material. HA has been used since 1981 and is composed of calcium-phosphate and is similar to native bone [17]. HA is well tolerated, can have overgrowth of mucosa, and resists infection and resorption [8]. HA prostheses are the only prostheses that currently do not require placement of cartilage to prevent extrusion (extrusion rate of 5%–10%). Problems with HA include difficulty in trimming (it requires use of a drill with irrigation) and risk of shattering. One must avoid placement of the HA prosthesis near the scutum to avoid osseointegration and fixation. Another criticism of these prostheses is that some HA prostheses are top-heavy and may tip over easily if not positioned securely.

HA has also been used in a malleable fashion as bone cement, instead of preformed prostheses [18,19]. Goebel and Jacob [19] used HA bone cement in 25 subjects in a variety of ossicular defects (such as incus erosion) and to assist with OCR (eg, to secure total or partial ossicular reconstruction prosthesis placement). Although average follow-up was only 11 months, mean air-bone gaps improved from 33 dB to 16 dB. Other types of bone cement (glass ionomer, silicate, and carboxylate) have also been used [20].

High-density polyethylene sponge is available as plastipore, which has been used since the 1970s and was the first alloplast sold commercially worldwide [3,5,8]. It requires the use of cartilage when in contact with the TM, to prevent extrusion. Plastipore is nonreactive and allows tissue ingrowth because of its porosity [5]. Thus, it is used most often as a shaft material in a hybrid or combination prosthesis (eg, with HA head). It is easy to trim and modify [8].

Titanium is another alloplastic material that is newer, increasingly used, and has shown much promise (Fig. 5). It is inert, light, and rigid [21]. Titanium was first used in 1993 [22]. It has been reported that visibility is improved over other types of prostheses because of fenestrations in the head [5,23]. Titanium requires cartilage to prevent extrusion but, overall, its success rate and extrusion rate (5%) approximates that of HA prostheses [5]. Schmerber and colleagues [24] reported on their experience with the Kurz titanium prostheses (both total and partial ossicular reconstruction prostheses) in 111 subjects. Overall, 66% of subjects had a postoperative air-bone gap of 20 dB or less. The investigators noted a significant difference in results between the total and partial ossicular reconstruction prostheses (25.2 dB versus 14.3 dB average air-bone gap, respectively). Two extrusions were noted at 17 and 20 months after surgery. The rate of sensorineural hearing loss was 3.6%.

Hybrid prostheses have been developed by some companies to minimize the disadvantages of each material, while capitalizing on their advantages. For example, HA is used typically as the head material to reduce risk of extrusion. Plastipore or titanium is used as shaft material for ease in trimming

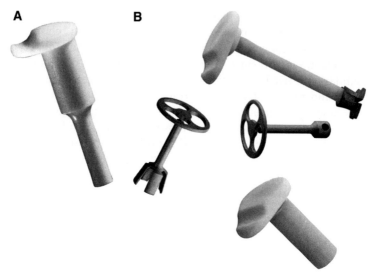

Fig. 5. Bojrab implant (*A*) and titanium prostheses (*B*). (Courtesy of Gyrus ACMI, Bartlett, TN; with permission.)

and modification. Unfortunately, because of HA comprising the head, these types of prostheses are top-heavy and have a risk of tipping over.

Staging of the ear

A benefit of staging the ear, particularly for the novice or occasional otologic surgeon, is that it simplifies decision making and allows a second chance to correct failures from the first surgery (eg, TM graft failure). Staging allows the separation of the surgical treatment of ear disease into two distinct phases. The primary goal is eradication of ear disease with creation of a clean, safe, and dry ear. The secondary goal is restoration of hearing. At the second stage, which is performed typically 6 to 12 months after the first surgery, one has a better appreciation of the final anatomic position the TM has taken, allowing for proper sizing of the prosthesis; this may also reduce the incidence of complications, such as erosion of the stapes footplate by a total ossicular reconstruction prosthesis or extrusion. The time also allows for regrowth of normal mucosa, while maintaining a middle ear space. The surgeon can also assess for recurrent or residual cholesteatoma.

Ideally, the plan for staging is discussed with the patient preoperatively, allowing for a change in decision making intraoperatively. The greater the amount of ear disease present, the higher the likelihood of needing staging. The only ossicular abnormality absolutely requiring staging (with COM) is stapes fixation due to otosclerosis or tympanosclerosis [8]. A stapedotomy or stapedectomy cannot be performed in the presence of active ear disease due to the risk of labryrinthitis and profound hearing loss.

Material can be placed in the middle ear space to prevent adhesion formation between the TM and mucosa of the middle ear, particularly over the cochlear promontory (especially if it is denuded). Materials used in staging include absorbable materials (such as gelfilm) and nonabsorbable sheeting (most commonly, silastic). Thick sheeting is preferred over thin sheeting to prevent displacement.

Preoperative consent

Before proceeding to the operating room, one must obtain a thorough preoperative consent, which includes discussing the risks of anesthesia and surgical procedures in general (eg, bleeding, pain, and so forth), and the risks of otologic procedures in specific (hearing loss or deafness, tinnitus, dizziness, ear drum perforation, facial nerve paralysis, otorrhea, taste changes, no guarantee of success). Other issues that may need to be discussed include the possible need for staging or revision procedures, placement of ventilation tubes, and recurrence of ear disease. In particular, the occasional otologic surgeon should realize that the success rates quoted in the literature for both primary and revision OCR are based on large surgical volumes and procedures performed by experienced surgeons. Expectations should be altered for less experienced surgeons.

Surgical technique

Proper surgical technique is key to successful OCR. Although potentially hard to quantify, one cannot overstate the importance of experience in the surgical treatment of ear disease and CHL. In revision surgery, the facial nerve may be dehiscent because of disease or prior procedures. Care is taken to prevent the prosthesis from touching the fallopian canal and causing facial paresis (or from touching the promontory or scutum, causing ankylosis) [3,25]. Thus, some surgeons prefer to perform revision ossiculoplasties only with the facial nerve monitor in place. In contradistinction, other surgeons prefer to perform revision ossiculoplasties with the patient under local anesthesia, to assess hearing improvement intraoperatively and allow for prosthesis adjustment if needed.

At the time of the revision procedure, the surgeon should find the reasons for the primary OCR failure. The incisions used for revision OCR depend on what is needed. If only middle ear work is needed (ie, placement of TM graft and prosthesis), a transcanal or endaural approach is used. If there is concern about disease involving the mastoid, then a postauricular incision is used, with the patient consented for mastoidectomy. A tympanomeatal flap is elevated and the middle ear is examined. If possible, the chorda tympani nerve is preserved. To avoid stapes subluxation, the surgeon should work along the stapes and oval window, parallel to the stapedial tendon.

Some surgeons use a laser for revision OCR cases to assist with lysing of adhesions, scar, and tympanosclerosis, and to minimize direct stapes movement and possible iatrogenic sensorineural hearing loss.

Some surgeons prefer only certain prostheses (ie, titanium or HA/plastipore). An argument can be made for becoming adept and familiar with one type of prosthesis, which can build surgical confidence and expertise. Alternatively, using different prostheses enhances one's repertoire and ability to use backup prostheses. Although gelfoam is used typically to stabilize the prosthesis intraoperatively, some surgeons use other bioabsorbable substances, such as fibrin glue or Sepragel, which is composed of hyaluronate and carboxymethylcellulose (Genzyme, Cambridge, Massachusetts) [26].

Results

The surgical goal is to significantly improve preoperative CHL, particularly in the speech frequencies, and to avoid the need for hearing aid placement for the long term. The audiometric goal is to achieve a postoperative air-conduction threshold of 30 dB, or an air-bone gap of 20 dB or less [5,27]. However, long-term data are limited, with only one randomized, prospective trial reported in the literature [5,28]. In addition, because of the numerous types of prostheses available, variety of surgical techniques, and criteria used to define success, it is difficult to truly compare results among prostheses.

The hearing results of revision OCR usually are not as good as those of primary OCR [21]. This difference is most likely because of several factors: severity of disease (requiring multiple surgeries), varied ossicular anatomy, and significant fibrosis and scar [8]. The prosthesis can fail to perform because of extrusion, displacement or slippage, fibrosis, inaccurate sizing, or resorption. Prosthesis extrusion can occur at any time postoperatively. Most extrusions heal spontaneously and in some patients hearing is maintained, even with the extrusion. The ossicular chain can contribute to failure by undergoing resorption or necrosis. If this occurs in the region of the stapes footplate, the patient is at risk of fistula formation, dizziness, and subsequent sensorineural hearing loss. If there is concern about footplate erosion at the time of revision OCR, perichondrium may be used before placement of the prosthesis. To a certain extent, all prostheses undergo long-term degradation in function. Thus, short-term results are typically better than long-term results. Colletti and colleagues [29] found that of 832 ossiculoplasties (partial and total ossicular reconstruction prostheses) reported, 77% had a CHL of 20 dB or less at 6 months. However, at 5 years of follow-up, only 42% had such a result. Yung [30] approximated a success rate at 5 years of two out of three for partial ossicular reconstruction prostheses and one out of three for total ossicular reconstruction prostheses.

Depending on the individual, an improved quality of life after revision OCR can be predicated on numerous factors, such as (1) being able to use the phone again on the affected ear, (2) noticing improved speech recognition in quiet and noise, (3) having improved directional hearing, (4) using a hearing aid, and (5) noticing improved appreciation for music. Patients tend to notice an improvement in hearing when symmetry is reached (ie, the worse hearing ear approximates the better hearing ear).

Regarding the future of revision OCR, Schuring [25] appropriately states that "...the future of ossiculoplasty will rest more on the solution of ancillary problems than on ossiculoplasty techniques. These troublesome ancillary problems include ETD, cholesteatoma control, mucosa regeneration, and fibrosis during the healing process. The self-correcting process of ossiculoplasty is an evolutionary process, and the small surgical steps taken are slowly incorporated into surgical principles."

References

[1] Wullstein H. The restoration of the function of the middle ear in chronic otitis media. Ann Otol Rhinol Laryngol 1956;65:1020–41.

[2] Zollner F. The principles of plastic surgery of the sound-conducting apparatus. J Laryngol Otol 1955;69:637–52.

[3] Merchant SN. Ossiculoplasty and tympanoplasty in chronic otitis media. In: Nadol JB Jr, McKenna MJ, editors. Surgery of the ear and temporal bone. 2nd edition. Philadelphia: Lippincott Williams & Wilkins; 2005. p. 305–24.

[4] Ruhl CM, Pensak ML. Role of aerating mastoidectomy in noncholesteatomatous chronic otitis media. Laryngoscope 1999;109:1924–7.

[5] Yung M. Long-term results of ossiculoplasty: reasons for surgical failure. Otol Neurotol 2006;27:20–6.

[6] Becvarovski Z, Kartush JM. Smoking and tympanoplasty: implications for prognosis and the Middle Ear Risk Index (MERI). Laryngoscope 2001;111(10):1806–11.

[7] Black B. Ossiculoplasty prognosis; the spite method of assessment. Am J Otol 1992;13(6): 544–51.

[8] Daniels RL, Shelton C. Revision ossicular reconstruction. In: Carrasco VN, Pillsbury HC, editors. Revision otologic surgery. New York: Thieme; 1997. p. 22–42.

[9] Martin C, Timoshenko AP, Martin C, et al. Cartilage and tympanoplasty. Acta Otorhinolaryngol Belg 2004;58(4):143–9.

[10] Iurato S, Marioni G, Onofri M. Hearing results of ossiculoplasty in Austin-Kartush group A patients. Otol Neurotol 2001;22(2):140–4.

[11] Schwetschenau EL, Isaacson G. Ossiculoplasty in young children with the Appelbaum incudostapedial joint prosthesis. Laryngoscope 1999;109(10):1621–5.

[12] Mills RP. Critical evaluation of the "jigsaw" assembly for ossiculoplasty. Am J Otol 1996; 17(1):19–23.

[13] Romanet P, Duvillard C, Delouane M. Mastoid cortical bone grafts in ossiculoplasty Ann Otolaryngol Chir Cervicofac 2000 Mar;117(2):105–9.

[14] O'Reilly RC, Cass SP, Hirsch BE, et al. Ossiculoplasty using incus interposition: hearing results and analysis of the middle ear risk index. Otol Neurotol 2005;26:853–8.

[15] Cura O, Kriazli T, Oztop F. Can homograft ossicles still be used in ossiculoplasty? Rev Laryngol Otol Rhinol (Bord) 2000;121(2):87–90.

[16] Chiossone E. Homograft ossiculoplasty: long-term results. Am J Otol 1987;8(6):545–50.

[17] Grote J. Tympanoplasty with calcium phosphate. Arch Otol 1984;110:197–9.

[18] Babu S, Seidman MD. Ossicular reconstruction using bone cement. Otol Neurotol 2004; 25(2):98–101.

[19] Goebel JA, Jacob A. Use of Mimix hydroxyapatite bone cement for difficult ossicular recon-
     struction. Otolaryngol Head Neck Surg 2005;132(5):727–34.
[20] Bayazit YA, Ozer E, Kanlikama M, et al. Bone cement ossiculoplasty: incus to stapes versus
     malleus to stapes cement bridge. Otol Neurotol 2005;26:364–7.
[21] Martin AD, Harner SG. Ossicular reconstruction with titanium prosthesis. Laryngoscope
     2004;114(1):61–4.
[22] Dalchow CV, Grun D, Stupp HF. Reconstruction of the ossicular chain with titanium im-
     plants. Otolaryngol Head Neck Surg 2001;125:628–30.
[23] Maassen MM, Lowenheim H, Pfister M, et al. Surgical-handling properties of the titanium
     prosthesis in ossiculoplasty. Ear Nose Throat J 2005;84(3):142–4, 147–9.
[24] Schmerber S, et al. Hearing results with the titanium ossicular replacement prostheses. Eur
     Arch Otorhinolaryngol 2005;(epublished ahead of print).
[25] Schuring AG. Ossiculoplasty with semibiologic and composite prostheses. Otolaryngol Clin
     North Am 1994;27(4):747–57.
[26] Shatkovskaya NY, Soushko YA, Veremeyenko KN, et al. Autofibrin glue compound and its
     utilization during reconstructive operations on the ear. Rev Laryngol Otol Rhinol (Bord)
     1999;120(1):53–6.
[27] Goode RL. Acoustical aspect of chronic ear surgery. 2nd edition. Rochester, MN: 1987.
[28] Mangham CA, Lindeman RC. Ceravital versus Plastipore in tympanoplasty: a randomized
     prospective trial. Ann Otol Rhinol Laryngol 1990;99:112–6.
[29] Colletti V, Fiorino FG, Sittoni V. Minisculptured ossicle grafts versus implants: long-term
     results. Am J Otol 1987;8:553–9.
[30] Yung MW. Literature review of alloplastic materials in ossiculoplasty. J Laryngol Otol 2003;
     117:431–6.

**ELSEVIER
SAUNDERS**

Otolaryngol Clin N Am
39 (2006) 713–721

OTOLARYNGOLOGIC
CLINICS
OF NORTH AMERICA

Endolymphatic Sac Revision for Recurrent Intractable Meniere's Disease

Michael M. Paparella, MD

*Minnesota Ear, Head and Neck Clinic, 701 25th Avenue South,
Suite 200, Minneapolis, MN 55454, USA*

In earlier publications, we described the etiology of Meniere's disease as based on multifactorial inheritance. Clinical evidence has accumulated since that first publication to support that initial concept strongly [1]. Genetic factors lead to obstructive anomalies, including a hypopneumatized mastoid, medial and anteriorly displaced sigmoid sinus, hypoplastic vestibular aqueduct and endolymphatic sac, reduction or absence of Trautmann's triangle (a key consideration relating to cause and treatment), and lack of development of the aditus ad antrum and adjacent suprapyramidal (facial) recess. Besides these intrinsic anomalies, extrinsic factors (diseases) can contribute concomitantly to the cause of Meniere's disease, factors such as otosclerosis, chronic inactive otitis media and chronic mastoiditis, trauma, and syphilis [1].

We described the pathogenesis of Meniere's disease to include malabsorption of the endolymphatic duct and sac and described attacks of Meniere's (cochlear and vestibular) as caused by chemical (labyrinthine membrane leaks and ruptures) and microphysical phenomena. In 1871, 10 years after Meniere described the disease that bears his name, Knapp referred to this disease as "glaucoma of the inner ear." In 1927, Michel Portmann Sr first described surgery on the endolymphatic sac for "glaucoma" of the inner ear. I find this analogy to continue to be valid, appropriate, and useful, especially when explaining the disease and its treatment options to patients. A treatment analogy also can be drawn. Ophthalmologic surgeons would apply drainage procedures for glaucoma, not destructive procedures. Similarly, we should consider conservative function preserving "drainage" procedures before considering destructive procedures for intractable Meniere's disease.

E-mail address: papar001@umn.edu

Considering the fact that the cause of intractable Meniere's disease is multifactorial inheritance and that its pathogenesis includes endolymphatic malabsorption leading to the glaucoma-like condition of the inner ear, among other studies and observations I have learned the most about the natural progression of Meniere's disease from revisions of enhancement surgery on the endolymphatic sac.

Clinical description

Meniere's disease is a clinical entity that can occur only in humans, although endolymphatic hydrops can be induced experimentally in animals. To understand its pathogenesis, it is important to study its natural history. With endolymphatic sac revisional surgery, we have a unique opportunity to let the disease evolve, intervene surgically with endolymphatic sac enhancement (ESE) for intractable Meniere's disease, and then later, if indicated, counteract further developments surgically to ameliorate cochlear and vestibular symptoms with revisional procedures. We get an opportunity to do just that in surgical revision for recurrent Meniere's disease after an initially good result of surgical enhancement of the endolymphatic sac years earlier. ESE helps to avoid destructive procedures, and revision has restored health to many patients. In the process revision also has provided the best opportunity for us to understand and observe the pathogenesis of Meniere's disease.

The first requirement in treating patients with progressive Meniere's disease who have intractable recurrent vertigo, deafness, or both involves medical and psychological support. If the intractable condition persists despite medical treatment, surgical enhancement may be required, and ESE is a relatively safe procedure that provides an opportunity to reverse conditions likely to cause hydrops (eg, malabsorption of endolymph) that favor the pathogenesis of Meniere's disease. We try to avoid labyrinthectomy because in the future these patients may be able to use a cochlear implant, an important consideration in a condition sometimes eventually susceptible to complete bilateral deafness.

Sometimes ESE produces excellent results that last for 3 or 4 years or more, but then vertigo, deafness, or other clinical symptoms may recur. We discuss with patients the option of surgical revision of the ESE. In the past we also offered the option of vestibular neurectomy when the original ESE failed, but only one of our patients has required vestibular nerve resection to date. In patients who choose revisional surgery we commonly see and correct further findings intraoperatively (extrasaccular fibrosis, osteoneogenesis, and aditus block), which causes symptoms to diminish or disappear after the revision, sometimes dramatically. Most patients do obtain decrease in or absence of their recurrent symptoms, and surgeons also gain intraoperative insights in this opportunity to study the pathogenesis that is unique, because Meniere's disease in humans is only observable in vivo.

Clinical study

Taking all their cases of revision of ESE between July 1982 and July 1986 that had at least 2 years of follow-up, Drs. Michael Paparella and Hamed Sajjadi assessed the patients' charts. There were 26 revisions, an incidence of 7%, although many of the original ESEs had been performed years earlier (before 1982), and the overall percentage of revision within that 4-year period was only 4%. All patients had a good result from their first endolymphatic sac procedure (loss of vertigo and retention of hearing), but symptoms gradually redeveloped over months and years. In the 26 revisions, the asymptomatic period ranged from 6 months to 11 years (average, 2.6 years). Two patients had sudden recurrence of vertigo and hearing loss—one patient 2.5 years after the ESE and the other 3.5 years after ESE. Another patient with bilateral Meniere's disease required one revision on the left ear and three revisions on the right ear, at the patient's request [2].

Reasons patients requested revision of their surgery included recurrent vertigo and hearing loss (in 22 patients) and hearing loss alone (in 4 patients). Another 2 patients underwent revisions during this period because of immediate postoperative infection of the wound along with copious granulation tissue and aditus block in the mastoid cavity, but those two cases are not included in this discussion. Intraoperative findings in each of the 26 revisions included osteoneogenesis and scar tissue near the endolymphatic sac. New bone was formed mostly from the adjacent lateral sinus and from within the infralabyrinthine cell tract. In some of these patients, removal of bone and decompression of the area in the original ESE had been insufficiently wide [2].

Copious scar tissue was seen routinely at revisional surgery, contiguous with the inferior margin of the wound and near the mastoid tip, always extrasaccular, not invading the lumen of the endolymphatic sac. Possibly this occurrence was caused by our method of making a small opening in the sac below the solid bony angle, but we also revised some cases in which the original procedure had been performed by other surgeons who did open the sac to the mastoid cavity. In six patients who later developed copious scar tissue, the initial procedure included grafting using temporalis fascia, which was performed routinely in those years. We discontinued this type of grafting in 1983 because of the findings we saw upon revision [2].

When we removed Silastic (Invotec International Inc., Jacksonville, Florida) from the sac, we observed that in every case it had a strong yellow discoloration, which suggested transudation of extracellular fluid. We have performed thousands of tympanoplasties and tympanomastoid procedures and routinely used Silastic in the middle ear, and we have seen this strong yellow discoloration in none of those thousands of procedures in the middle ear, but we routinely see it in revision of ESE procedures. Among other findings, this finding provides insight into the pathogenesis of Meniere's disease. Epithelium in the lumen in revised ESEs was shiny and intact. In 2 patients, the aditus ad antrum was completely obstructed and in 11 patients it was partially obstructed, and there was more tissue formed in the mastoid cavity. Two patients showed a bony shelf (operculum, an anatomic variant) on the subdural side that obviated decompression at that site [2].

Recurrence of hearing loss only was the reason for election of revision for 4 patients who did not have vertigo; in 3 patients, hearing improved discrimination an average of 24% and speech reception threshold 16 dB on average, although there was no change in the fourth patient. The remaining 22 patients elected revision for recurrence of hearing loss and vertigo; in 9 patients, hearing stayed the same, but 13 gained improved hearing, on average a 20% increase in discrimination and 18 dB in speech reception threshold. The recurrence of hearing loss and vertigo had occurred suddenly—years after the initial procedure—in 2 patients in whom we performed exploratory tympanotomy with the revision of the ESE to investigate whether the sudden deafness might have been caused by perilymphatic fistula. Drainage of perilymph was seen at the round window in 1 patient and was strongly suggested in the other patient, so we grafted the round windows, and both patients achieved improved hearing after revision. All but 1 of these 22 had significant improvement of vertigo. It was eliminated in 12 patients and substantially controlled in 9. One patient did require sectioning of the vestibular nerve [2].

Technique

Our technique for ESE has been modified somewhat on the basis of these findings from revisions of the procedure. As described elsewhere [3], our clinic treats the wound differently. Because in some cases there were problems with postoperative infection of the wound, currently an elliptical incision is made three fourths of an inch behind the postauricular crease and ends posterior to the mastoid tip inferiorly so that the line of incision does not cross the open mastoid cavity. We elevate skin with attached periosteum. If the postauricular skin contains thick dermis, as it often does in these patients, we thin it with plastic scissors to discourage later fibroblastic invasion from the site into a hypoplastic mastoid. This procedure is often a routine adjunct to revision of ESE procedures. We finish the procedure with meticulous removal of debris from the wound and control of all subcutaneous bleeders to prevent entry into the mastoid of blood, which can promote scarring and formation of granulation tissue. We carefully close the wound with subcutaneous sutures and surgical clips to close the skin.

As a second modification, we perform a complete mastoidectomy with wide exposure. We usually find the sac anterior and inferior to the posteroinferior semicircular canal. Routinely, the lateral (sigmoid) sinus is abnormally located more medially and anteriorly than usual, and we widely expose it and remove bone over it. We noticed that in some revisions the lateral sinus had not been as widely decompressed in the initial ESE as it should have been; bone remained in a remote region that did not allow effective decompression of the dura and contiguous sac. Such bone from the lateral sinus can create osteoneogenesis that grows toward the sac, so try not to leave bone on the adjacent lateral sinus or dura.

Third, we modified the procedure to open the aditus widely contiguous with the suprapyramidal or facial recess not only to expose the incus and its fossa incudis (an important landmark) but also to encourage good aeration between middle ear and mastoid cavity. Bone dust regularly accumulates near the oval window and with direct visualization and irrigation must be removed to prevent fixation of the stapes and a postoperative conductive hearing loss.

To ensure wide decompression, we remove bone generally in an exaggerated manner over Trautmann's triangle and over the adjacent lateral sinus to decompress the lateral sinus contiguous with the dura of the posterior cranial fossa (containing the sac). We enhance this decompression by using coiled spacers made of Silastic to act as loose springs that separate tight dura from the bone of the solid angle. We no longer cover the sac with fascia but rather with an "apron" of Silastic to protect against fibroblastic invasion. We shape and coil a Silastic T-strut (small, medium, or large) within the lumen of the sac and use the spacers to decompress the dura above and below the sac as far as possible. As we open the sac widely under the solid angle, we use Silastic spacers under the solid angle (bony shelf) to contain the environment to this region rather than let it extend toward the open mastoid cavity.

We routinely place a myringotomy and ventilation tube in the anterior tympanic membrane to promote healing, drainage, and ventilation, help avoid otitis media (sometimes related to flying), and help aerate the mastoid to try to discourage aditus block syndrome, osteoneogenesis, and formation of fibrous tissue in the mastoid during postoperative years.

In approximately 7% to 8% of patients, the dura contiguous with the endolymphatic sac in Trautmann's triangle is delicate and thin, and drainage of cerebrospinal fluid results, sometimes simply from carefully removing bone from the dura. In some instances the bone is inherently attached with the dura and cannot be separated. In these cases we pack the mastoid tightly with dry gelfoam, and with no heavy exercise or lifting and with elevation of the head, the patient heals without further treatment. In more than 3500 patients to date who have received ESE, only a handful of patients—a minor fraction of 1%—required a lumbar drain or a revisional procedure to graft and stop the drainage of cerebrospinal fluid.

Finally, we observed that it has been helpful to saturate and perfuse the endolymphatic sac with gentamicin, including exposure of the round window to gentamicin, for 7 to 8 minutes during revisional procedures in selected patients who have severe hearing loss but who need clinical elimination of vertigo.

Discussion

*Clinical implications of revisions of endolymphatic sac
enhancement procedures*

Because most patients already have had good primary results from
an ESE, revisions can result in elimination or improvement of vertigo and
improvement in hearing, with a greater likelihood of success than from
the initial procedure. Years later, surgical scar tissue and iatrogenic osteoneogenesis may recreate the pathogenic conditions so that correction of
the secondary lesions provides a good opportunity for beneficial results. Primary findings to be corrected at the time of revision may include formation
of extrasaccular bone and fibrous tissue, aditus block, tight dura near the
sac, and yellowed Silastic within and near the sac.

After the revision, hearing was found to be significantly better, twice as
good in 62% of our patients (increasing at least 15 dB in speech reception
threshold and 15% in speech discrimination), whereas the initial ESE produced significantly better hearing in only 30% to 40%. Some patients
achieved dramatic restoration of hearing after revision, going from deafness
to useful hearing. In three of four such patients there was improvement in
recurrent hearing loss that occurred alone without vertigo. Of patients
who had hearing loss and vertigo, 95% achieved control or elimination of
vertigo after revision of the ESE. In two patients in whom an initially
good ESE suddenly reverted to hearing loss, vertigo, or both, we identified
and treated an associated perilymphatic fistula of the round window.

This study found risks from revision of ESE to be minimal, and results
were gratifying. All but one patient continue to do well with this conservative therapy, and only one patient required intracranial vestibular nerve section. This finding indicates that patients with good results from ESE who
later develop delayed recurrence of vertigo or hearing loss can be considered
for revisions or even repeated revisions of ESE. If the primary problem remains to be vertigo, then retrolabyrinthine vestibular nerve section (in cases
of normal or near-normal hearing), surgical labyrinthectomy (in cases of
useless hearing while the opposite ear has normal hearing), or chemical ablation (intratympanic gentamicin, a first, best option if revision fails) still
can be considered. Even then, we make every effort to avoid these destructive procedures because a significant number of patients who have Meniere's
disease eventually develop bilateral deafness. If a surgical labyrinthectomy
has been performed, it may compromise consideration of a cochlear implant
that may be needed in the future. While examining a relatively limited number of patients since the 4-year period reported in our study, we have seen
many other patients demonstrate similar findings. Better results, in fact,
may be obtained in revision than in initial ESE.

Currently throughout the medical literature there has been emphasis on
using intratympanic gentamicin to treat patients who have intractable

vertigo caused by Meniere's disease. This approach is not new, because Dr. Hanson, Chief of the Veterans' Administration Hospitals in the mid-1940s, used ototoxic drugs to treat Meniere's disease, and the approach was later popularized by Drs. Fowler Sr. and Fowler Jr. of Columbia University and Dr. Schuknecht from the 1950s onward. I had the opportunity to treat many patients decades ago with intratympanic streptomycin or gentamicin, particularly parenterally induced streptomycin. Our studies clearly indicated that it is a cochleotoxic and vestibulotoxic drug, even if it does not demonstrate discernible hearing loss with routine audiometry.

The cochlear duct is approximately 31 mm long in humans, which means that the basal turn, where the high frequencies are located, approximates one third to one half of the length of the scala media or cochlear duct. We find in our otopathologic studies that the basal turn routinely shows damage to the hair cells of the organ of Corti after administration of ototoxic drugs, and we know that there is a high incidence of hearing loss in patients even when routine measurable behavioral audiometry is used. Routine behavioral audiometry does not measure the basal turn and only measures bone conduction up to 4000 cps. For this reason we believe that conservative treatment of patients who have Meniere's disease—first medical treatment, then sac enhancement, and then revision of the ESE years later if necessary—is still the best process. Whether chemical or surgical labyrinthectomy is involved, these procedures are destructive to the cochlear and vestibular labyrinth. Although we use them, we use them as "court of last resort" and have found that we can preserve hearing and save the hearing in patients who have Meniere's disease, particularly bilateral Meniere's disease, with greater success than using techniques destructive to the inner ear. Vestibular neurectomy still plays a role but a markedly diminished role compared with that in former years. A simple logical observation by my patients surmises that "once you destroy something, you cannot put it back."

Natural progression of pathogenesis for Meniere's disease and induced Meniere's disease

In revisions of ESE, each patient serves as his or her own control so that our observations intraoperatively in these revisions gain clinicians' insights into the nature, cause, pathogenesis, and treatment of Meniere's disease. There is a unique opportunity in studying conditions in these patients to follow the natural history of this disease, which in humans is seen only in vivo, so that we can make a diagnosis of intractable Meniere's disease and treat it with an ESE, only to have symptoms recur later when we can see the conditions that developed them. The ESE is a procedure designed to reverse conditions that seem to contribute to the fundamental pathogenic process of Meniere's disease, such as malabsorption of endolymph. Some patients (approximately 7%) have good results, typically for a few years or more after their initial ESE, but then become candidates for a revisional procedure when they experience delayed, gradual recurrence of symptoms with the associated role of iatrogenic inducement. We can observe these conditions intraoperatively, correct them, and observe beneficial results in most of these revisions. The following hypothesis describes the rationale for the efficacy of ESE and endolymphatic sac revision.

Hypothesis concerning decompression

Because of pathologic, genetically induced anatomic abnormalities, patients who have Meniere's disease have a tight endolymphatic sac and contiguous dura and a medially and anteriorly displaced lateral sinus. In treating the condition surgically, this abnormality requires complete simple mastoidectomy, wide removal of bone from over Trautmann's triangle and the lateral sinus, and decompression of dura in Trautmann's triangle and beneath the solid angle. We enhance decompression using Silastic T-struts to enlarge the lumen and use Silastic spacers to loosen dura from bone above and below the sac. The hypothesis is that decompression is the most important surgical contribution to counteracting the important pathogenic mechanism of obstruction of a tightened, restricted sac and dura.

Hypothesis concerning transudation and osmotic pull

In an ear with Meniere's disease, an osmotic pressure differential is created between the extracellular milieu within and near the sac (high in sodium) and endolymph on the other side of the vestibular aqueduct (high in potassium). Transudate produced in this flow turns Silastic that was placed in the sac at initial ESE yellow by the time of revisional surgery. The environment that affects it is not in the mastoid cavity but rather lies between bone and dura. One may compare Silastic retrieved from the middle ear routinely (eg, in thousands of surgical revisions of tympanoplasty over the years), which retains its original clear color.

Hypothesis concerning passive diffusion of endolymph and enlargement of the endolymphatic sac

By enlarging the saccular lumen and placing Silastic (alloplastic) T-struts within the lumen, the revisional surgery provides surfaces against which nanoliters of endolymph can transgress passively. The Silastic T-strut acts as a wick exiting the sac to lie under bone, not in the mastoid cavity.

Hypothesis concerning altered blood supply and immune characteristics

Collateral blood supply may be encouraged by manipulating the blood supply around the sac. We isolate the region using a Silastic "apron" to separate the sac from the mastoid cavity to help prevent fibroblastic invasion. Either ESE or its revision also may alter immune properties within the sac.

Summary

Endolymphatic sac revision after an initially successful ESE procedure has been found to have a useful role for patients who have recurrent intractable Meniere's disease. Most of these patients have benefited from revisional surgery with loss or control of vertigo, retention or improvement of hearing, and improvement of symptoms of pressure, tinnitus, and inability to tolerate loudness.

In addition to its clinical efficacy, endolymphatic sac revision provides the best opportunity to observe objective findings (eg, fibroblastic and osteogenetic invasion, an obstructed, tight sac and contiguous dura, and marked yellow discoloration of previously placed Silastic T-struts and spacers) that enhance a visible observation and understanding of the pathogenesis over time. Correction of these pathologic findings in the region of Trautmann's triangle seems to improve malabsorption and dysfunction in the endolymphatic sac. Endolymphatic sac enhancements and revisional procedures correct a patient's symptoms by reversing (affecting) the role of the endolymphatic sac in the pathogenesis of Meniere's disease.

References

[1] Paparella MM. The cause (multifactorial inheritance) and pathogenesis (malabsorption of endolymph) of Meniere's disease and its symptoms (mechanical and chemical). Acta Otolaryngol 1985;99(3–4):445–51.
[2] Paparella MM, Sajjadi H. Endolymphatic sac revision for recurrent Meniere's disease. Am J Otol 1988;9(6):441–7.
[3] Paparella MM. Endolymphatic sac procedures. In: Brackmann DE, Shelton C, Arriaga MA, editors. Otologic surgery. 2nd edition. Philadelphia: WB Saunders; 2001. p. 371–84.

ELSEVIER
SAUNDERS

Otolaryngol Clin N Am
39 (2006) 723–740

OTOLARYNGOLOGIC
CLINICS
OF NORTH AMERICA

Revision Mastoidectomy

Joseph B. Nadol Jr, MD[a,b]

[a]*Department of Otology and Laryngology, Harvard Medical School, Boston, MA, USA*
[b]*Department of Otolaryngology, Massachusetts Eye and Ear Infirmary,*
243 Charles St., Boston, MA 02114, USA

The first three priorities in surgery for chronic otitis media are (1) the elimination of progressive disease to produce a safe and dry ear, (2) modification of the anatomy of the tympanomastoid compartment to prevent recurrent disease, and (3) reconstruction of the hearing mechanism. The indications for revision following mastoidectomy for chronic otitis media thus involve failure to achieve any of these goals, including recurrent cholesteatoma, recurrent suppuration, recurrent perforation, or recurrent or residual conductive hearing loss. The focus of this article is the management of recurrent cholesteatoma or suppuration; that is, failure to achieve either of the first two priorities.

The published failure rates for primary mastoidectomy for chronic suppurative otitis media vary widely, ranging from 3% to 26%, or more [1–12]. The factors responsible for surgical failure are multiple, and include the subcategory of disease, the anatomic consequences of primary surgery, or a combination of the original disease process and the surgical approach selected. For example, chronic otitis media with cholesteatoma treated with canal wall up mastoidectomy has been recognized as having a high rate of residual and recurrent cholesteatoma, in the range of 29% or higher [4,7,11], whereas other investigators [13] have suggested that chronic otitis media without cholesteatoma, but with granulation tissue, is more difficult to control over the long-term than cholesteatoma, perhaps because of more widespread disease.

Given the wide spectrum of disease included in the term "chronic otitis media," and the number of surgical procedures that may be used to address this disorder, the development of a successful strategy for revision mastoidectomy requires a clear and logical nomenclature, both for diagnostic

E-mail address: joseph_nadol@meei.harvard.edu

categories and surgical procedures, and an understanding of the pertinent histopathology of chronic active otitis media that may influence the selection or success of the surgical procedure.

Diagnostic categories of chronic otitis media

The author's preference for categorization of various subtypes of chronic otitis media is shown in Box 1. Thus, chronic active otitis media includes subtypes with and without cholesteatoma, whereas chronic inactive otitis media implies no evidence of either cholesteatoma or ongoing suppuration. Even within categories of chronic otitis media, including cholesteatoma, there exist important distinctions that may influence the selection of a successful management strategy. For example, a small cholesteatoma of the epitympanum without otorrhea may be managed very successfully with a limited surgical procedure, such as an anterior atticotomy. On the other hand, a cholesteatoma of similar location and size, but with continuous suppuration, implies much more widespread involvement of the tympano-mastoid compartment, with sequestration of disease and resultant suppuration, which requires a much more extensive surgical procedure for successful control.

In chronic active otitis media without cholesteatoma, continuous otorrhea implies significant sequestration of disease, or unexenterated cells that are likely to require revision surgery, whereas intermittent otorrhea may be due to simple mechanical problems, an unstable epithelium, or superinfection, which may be managed medically or with minor surgical procedures, such as split thickness skin grafting of the mastoid bowl.

Box 1. Diagnostic categories of COM (primary or recurrent)

I. Chronic active otitis media
A. With cholesteatoma
   Without otorrhea
   With otorrhea
B. Without cholesteatoma
   With continuous otorrhea
   With intermittent otorrhea

II. Chronic inactive otitis media
With retraction pocket
With perforation
With ossicular resorption or fixation
With adhesive otitis media

Surgical procedures for chronic otitis media

Surgical procedures for chronic otitis media are shown in Box 2. A number of surgical decisions must be made from the beginning to the end of any surgical procedure for chronic active otitis media, including those about incisions, osseous approaches, and modifications both to soft tissue and to the bony anatomy of the temporal bone. Appropriate surgical planning requires a decision in each of these areas to create a unique surgical plan, based on the surgeon's evaluation of the extent of recurrent chronic otitis media and the reasons for previous surgical failure. Although there are a number of histopathologic findings in chronic suppurative otitis media that influence the surgical approach and the success of ossicular reconstruction, the emphasis here is to review examples of histopathology that may influence the surgical approach and the success in management of progressive disease, either cholesteatoma or suppuration.

As a biologic response to chronic otitis media, both sclerosing and osteoresorptive processes may be found, with or without cholesteatoma. Familiarity with these processes helps the surgeon prepare for a revision surgical

---

Box 2. Nomenclature for surgical management of COM

Incisions
Transmeatal
Endaural
Postauricular

Osseous approaches
Atticotomy
Anterior
Anterior-posterior
Canal wall up tympanomastoidectomy
Canal wall down mastoidectomy
Canal wall down mastoidectomy with reconstruction of posterior
　canal wall

Modifications
Soft tissue
　Meatoplasty
　Obliterative techniques
　Grafting
　• Split thickness skin graft
　• Fascia
　• Cartilage
Osseous
　• Canalplasty

procedure. Modern imaging studies, principally CT scan of the temporal bone, also assist the surgeon in this evaluation.

Sclerosing processes

Fibrocystic sclerosis

As a result of chronic suppuration and granulation tissue, fibrous tissue may be deposited in the submucosal plane, causing progressive sequestration and loculation of previously pneumatized spaces of the middle ear and mastoid (Fig. 1). This process may lead to clinically identifiable entities, such as "aditus block" [14,15]. Fibrocystic sclerosis may also exacerbate dysfunction of the eustachian tube and limit the potential for reconstructive procedures for hearing, when the process involves either the oval or round window areas. The presence of fibrocystic sclerosis often is interpreted on radiographic imaging as "soft tissue opacification" of the middle ear or mastoid.

Fibro-osseous sclerosis

The reparative process in chronic active otitis media also includes the deposition of new bone, which, like fibrocystic sclerosis, may result in obstruction and loculation of disease (Fig. 2). Often, the presence of fibro-osseous sclerosis is detected on radiographic imaging of the temporal bone and is identified by the radiologist as a "poorly pneumatized" or "sclerotic" mastoid. Fibro-osseous sclerosis may also interfere with identification of critical landmarks in chronic ear surgery and may impede complete exenteration of infected mastoid cells.

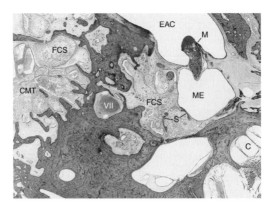

Fig. 1. Fibrocystic sclerosis of the middle ear and mastoid in the left ear of a patient with chronic otitis media. In the middle ear, the fibrocystic sclerosis surrounds the stapes superstructure. C, cochlea; CMT, mastoid; EAC, external auditory canal; FCS, fibrocystic sclerosis; M, manubrium; ME, middle ear ; VII, facial nerve; S, stapes superstructure.

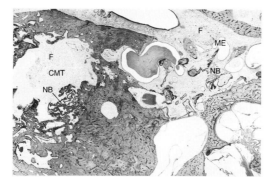

Fig. 2. Fibro-osseous sclerosis. Fibrous tissue (F) and new bone (NB) fill much of the central mastoid track (CMT) and middle ear (ME) in the left ear of a patient with chronic otitis media.

Osteoresorptive processes

Rarifying osteitis

Osteoclastic resorption of bone within the mastoid, otic capsule, or ossicles may occur, even in the absence of osteomyelitis, and may accompany chronic active otitis media with or without cholesteatoma (Fig. 3). It may lead to either limited or broad exposure of the dura of the middle or posterior cranial fossa; dehiscences of the otic capsule, resulting in labyrinthine fistulas (Fig. 4); or extensive exposure of the facial nerve, usually in the horizontal and first portion of the descending segments. A hint as to the presence of rarifying osteitis can be detected on radiologic imaging of the temporal bone, and is described by radiologists in various terms, such as "bony resorption" or "presence of an osteolytic process."

The revision surgeon is well served by the use of a diagnostic algorithm for self-categorization of the recurrent disease, and the development of a rational medical and surgical approach to management. Key elements include clinical evaluation, bacteriology, radiologic imaging, and analysis of previous surgical failure.

Clinical evaluation

Clinical evaluation includes a thorough and specific otologic history and otoscopic examination. The otologist may wish to develop a checklist similar to the process used by an airline pilot in preparation for flight. Elements of the checklist and key elements of both history and examination are provided in Box 3. Pertinent elements of the history of chronic otitis media include characterization and onset of the original disease process; details, as best can be determined, of prior otologic surgery; and a detailed description of the onset and characterization of recurrent symptoms. For example, if there is otorrhea, is it constant or intermittent? Is there pain or hearing loss, or are there facial nerve or other cranial neuropathies or vestibular

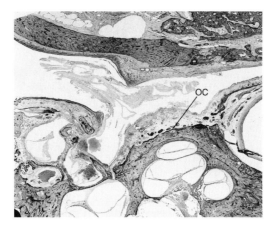

Fig. 3. Rarifying osteitis. As a consequence of chronic otitis media, the otic capsule (OC) was partially resorbed.

symptoms? In addition, pertinent medical history, including diabetes, immunosuppression, or allergic rhinosinusitis, should be documented.

The otologic examination is critical and in most cases requires an examining binocular microscope and documentation, either photodocumentation or the creation of detailed drawings of the findings and pertinent anatomy. For example, is there cholesteatoma or simply evidence for granulation? Is there drainage? Is the recurrence in the middle ear and is the previous mastoid bowl perfectly dry? Alternatively, is it the epicenter of disease in the mastoid and, if so, in what location, such as sinodural angle, tegmen, or mastoid tip? The anatomic consequences resulting from the first surgical procedure should be evaluated carefully, including the adequacy of the external auditory meatus, status of the posterior canal wall, status of the facial

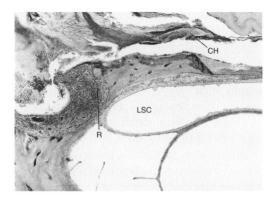

Fig. 4. Rarifying osteitis of the vestibular labyrinth. In this left ear, with chronic otitis media and cholesteatoma (CH), there is partial resorption (R) of the bone overlying the lateral semicircular canal (LSC).

Box 3. Evaluation algorithm for chronic active otitis media

I. Clinical evaluation
A. History
- Onset and characterization of initial symptoms
- Details of prior otologic surgery
- Onset and characterization of recurrent symptoms (eg, otorrhea, constant or intermittent), pain, hearing loss, cranial neuropathy, vestibular symptoms
- Pertinent general medical history (eg, diabetes, immunosuppression, allergic rhinosinusitis)
B. Otologic exam
- Documentation (photo, drawings of pertinent anatomy)
- Location of active disease (middle ear? mastoid?)
- Anatomic factors (eg, adequacy of meatus, status of posterior canal wall, facial ridge, residual cells, mastoid tip)

II. Bacteriology
III. Radiologic imaging
IV. Analysis of reasons for previous surgical failure

---

ridge, evaluation of residual mastoid cells, and access for otologic hygiene in such areas as the sinodural angle or mastoid tip.

In cases in which otorrhea is an important element of the disease process, culture and sensitivity of pathogens may play a significant role. For example, chronic suppurative otitis media, particularly following canal wall down procedures, may include several simultaneous pathogens, such as anaerobic organisms [16,17], and commonly used otologic topical antibiotics, in general, have poor anaerobic coverage. In the absence of cholesteatoma, medical management of chronic suppurative otitis media may be considered, at least initially [18].

Radiologic imaging

Radiologic imaging, principally CT, MRI, and magnetic resonance angiography, may provide important information to guide the revision surgery. For example, CT scanning may demonstrate the location of unexenterated and sequestrated cells in the hypotympanum (Fig. 5) or the presence of an unanticipated disease beyond the usual confines of the mastoid (Figs. 6 and 7), and may aid in the analysis of the reasons for previous surgical failure.

The information achieved by clinical evaluation, bacteriology, and radiologic imaging is integrated to form an educated opinion concerning the

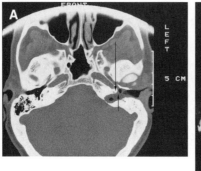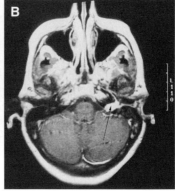

Fig. 5. Hypotympanic involvement by chronic otitis media of the left ear. (*A*) The CT scan demonstrated erosion of the hypotympanic cell system (*short arrow*). A resultant cochlear fistula (*long arrow*) caused profound sensorineural hearing loss. (*B*) The MR scan with gadolinium enhancement demonstrated enhancing granulation tissue in the hypotympanum (*arrow*). (*From* Nadol JB, McKenna MJ. Surgery of the ear and temporal bone. 2nd edition. Philadelphia: Lippincott, Williams and Wilkins; 2005; with permission.)

reasons for previous mastoid surgery failure; this will allow establishment of a rational treatment algorithm. Examples of common scenarios and analysis of previous surgical failure are shown in Box 4. It is useful to separate surgical failures into early failures, which in large part represent residual disease, and late failures, which may imply recurrent disease.

The typical scenarios may differ for early and late failures, based on the previous surgical approach. Thus, a common cause for surgical failure in

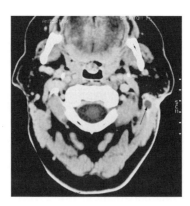

Fig. 6. A cholesteatoma (*arrow*) is shown in the soft tissue inferior to the left mastoid tip in this 65-year-old man who underwent multiple revision surgical procedures for chronic otitis media complicated by neck abscesses. A cholesteatoma had broken through the mastoid cortex and extended to the neck. This component of the cholesteatoma was overlooked in multiple revision procedures until demonstrated on this CT before the final surgical procedure. (*From* Nadol JB, McKenna MJ. Surgery of the ear and temporal bone. 2nd edition. Philadelphia: Lippincott, Williams and Wilkins; 2005; with permission.)

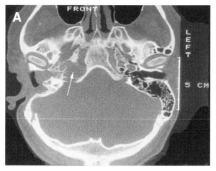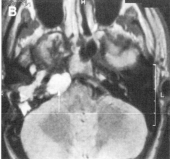

Fig. 7. Extension of chronic otitis media from the mastoid to the petrous apex in a patient who underwent multiple revision procedures for chronic otitis media. The CT scan (*A*) and MRI (*B*) demonstrated a large cyst of the petrous apex (*arrow*) that was in direct continuity with the infected tympanomastoid air cell system by way of the infralabyrinthine (hypotympanic) cells. This infected cyst served as a reservoir for continued otorrhea for many years. (*From* Nadol JB, McKenna MJ. Surgery of the ear and temporal bone. 2nd edition. Philadelphia: Lippincott, Williams and Wilkins; 2005; with permission.)

canal wall up tympanomastoidectomy is failure to modify the anatomy of the ear to render recurrence less likely. Examples include recurrent attic retraction or cholesteatoma, postoperative sequestration of the mastoid from the middle ear due to aditus block, or obstruction of the surgically created facial recess. In contrast, in canal wall down tympanomastoidectomy, more common causes of recurrent disease and late failure include obstruction; sequestration; and reinfection of residual air cells, particularly in the tegmen, sinodural angle, facial recess mastoid tip, or hypotympanum [19,20]. Over time, the meatus of the external ear canal may collapse or stenose because of inadequate meatoplasty, new bone formation, or anterior migration of the auricle. Inadequate lowering of the facial ridge or inadequate obliteration of exenterated cells may result in remucosalization, resequestration of disease, or inability to provide local hygiene. Nowhere is this concept better illustrated than in the problems faced in canal wall down fenestration cavities, which now have been largely abandoned for management of otosclerosis. In this procedure, a previous uninfected mastoid is partially exenterated, using a canal wall down approach, to allow hearing reconstruction. Unfortunately, an all-too-common complication of the fenestration procedure was the creation of a chronically draining mastoid bowl [21]. In such a case, the development of postoperative drainage must be attributed to the surgical procedure itself, rather than to recurrent disease (Fig. 8).

It is important to recognize the fundamental differences in surgical objectives in canal wall up versus canal wall down techniques. In both approaches, the initial surgical objectives are the same, namely to eliminate disease and to modify the anatomy to prevent recurrence. However, it is anticipated in the canal wall up procedure that remucosalization of the epitympanum and mastoid will result in a healthy, aerated cavity. In contrast,

---

Box 4. Algorithm for analysis of previous surgical failure for chronic active otitis media

I. Early failures

A. Both (canal wall up and canal wall down)
   Residual cholesteatoma
   Inadequate removal of sequestrated cells
   Unrecognized locus of disease
   • Hypotympanum
   • Sinus tympani
   • Petrous apex
   • Neck
   Unusual pathogen (eg, tuberculosis)

B. Canal wall down
   Stenosis, inaccessibility for postoperative aural hygiene
   Remucosalization of residual mastoid cells, particularly at tegmen and sinodural angle

II. Late failures

A. Both canal wall up and canal wall down
   Recurrent retraction or cholesteatoma

B. Canal wall up
   Recurrent aditus block or obstruction of surgically created facial recess

C. Canal wall down
   Meatal stenosis
   Inaccessibility for aural hygiene
   High facial ridge
   Inaccessible mastoid tip
   • New bone formation

---

in the canal wall down procedure, remucosalization and subsequent submucosal fibrosis may result in recurrent sequestration of disease and recurrent suppuration. In this sense, depending on aeration of the mastoid and adjacent areas, an adequate canal wall down procedure may be more difficult to accomplish than a canal wall up procedure.

Elements of successful revision surgery and special techniques for revision mastoid surgery

Success in creating a safe, dry ear and preventing recurrence is facilitated by the correct disease categorization and a correct and complete analysis of the reasons for previous surgical failure.

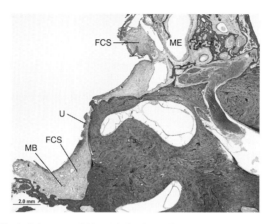

Fig. 8. Chronically draining mastoid bowl following a fenestration procedure. This patient underwent a fenestration procedure for otosclerosis at the age of 42 in the left ear and had chronic intermittent otorrhea until his death at age 63. There was chronic inflammation and ulceration (U) and fibrocystic sclerosis (FCS) in both the mastoid bowl (MB) and in the middle ear space (ME).

Informed consent for revision mastoidectomy for chronic otitis media

It is desirable to provide the patient preoperatively with as much detail as possible concerning the planned surgical procedure, based on evaluation and analysis. However, despite a thorough preoperative evaluation, not all elements of disease can be anticipated. As a result, there may be a need for intraoperative surgical judgment to modify the initially planned procedure. The proposed incisions or alternates, the extent of the surgical field, and the use of other materials, such as cartilage or skin grafts, should be discussed. Alternative therapeutic options, if any, should be disclosed. The risks of surgery to hearing, balance, and facial nerve function, and the risks of residual or recurrent disease, should be outlined.

Although obvious to the surgeon, it is not intuitively obvious to the patient that the healing phase following revision chronic otitis media may extend to weeks or even months. The patient should be informed that complete healing is not achieved with suture removal at 7 days, and that postoperative otologic follow-up, and even the possibility of a minor procedure, such as debridement or split thickness skin grafts, may be necessary. Failure to inform a patient of these facts may erode the patient's confidence in the therapy and commitment to the postoperative course.

The specific surgical procedures relevant to revision mastoid surgery may be divided easily into (1) procedures for complete removal of disease, and (2) modifications to either soft tissue or bone, in an effort to prevent a second or subsequent recurrence.

Complete removal of disease

Preoperative clinical evaluation to delineate the limits of disease is important in this regard. Surgical exposure is also a critical element. For example, although it is highly desirable to maintain the posterior canal wall, this is not always possible. In general, the most suitable cases for canal wall up mastoidectomy include those with a well-pneumatized mastoid, clinical evidence for good eustachian tube function, and limited atticoantral disease; and where there is the ability to preserve the tympanic membrane and ossicular chain. Relative contraindications include previous surgery for chronic active otitis media with extensive residual or recurrent disease; a poorly pneumatized and sclerotic mastoid; extensive granulation tissue; poor eustachian tube function; or the presence of otologic complications, such as facial nerve paresis or labyrinthine fistula. Canal wall down mastoidectomy may well be a better option where there is extensive disease; poorly pneumatized mastoid; presence of complications; clinical evidence of poor tubal function, ipsilaterally or bilaterally; and previous surgery leading to either residual or recurrent disease.

Surgical exposure

Limited middle ear disease may be managed by transmeatal or endaural incisions; however, in general, the postauricular incision is best suited for wide exposure and visualization of the disease process, including unanticipated findings. In an effort to prevent surgical injury to structures that may have been exposed by either the disease process or the previous surgical procedure, such as the dura of the middle or posterior cranial fossa, lateral venous sinus, or facial nerve, modification of the usual procedure is indicated. A somewhat longer postauricular incision allows identification of proper planes, and wider exposure. Beginning the surgical procedure both superior and posterior to the previous surgical field facilitates proper identification and avoidance of injury to these structures, and identification of surgical landmarks.

Generally, adhesions between musculofascial pedicles and bone are divided easily. In contrast, tight adherence between soft tissue and underlying structures strongly suggests adhesions between the soft tissue pedicle and underlying dura or other critical structures, such as the facial nerve. Usually, such adhesions then are cut sharply, rather than avulsed, in an effort to avoid injury.

Intraoperative monitoring of facial nerve function assists significantly in identifying the facial nerve in a previously surgically altered field, and provides an early warning system to identify maneuvers that may injure the nerve, such as dissection of pedicles from the nerve. In the presence of granulation tissue, particular attention should be paid to the mastoid tip, sinodural angle, tegmental cells, and hypotympanum (Fig. 9) [19,20]. Similarly, in chronic active otitis media with cholesteatoma and otorrhea,

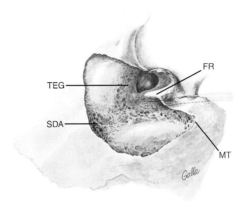

Fig. 9. An incomplete mastoidectomy (right ear). The facial ridge (FR) has not been lowered to the level of the nerve. In addition, there are many residual cells along the tegmen (TEG), in the sinodural angle (SDA), and in the mastoid tip (MT).

simple removal of the cholesteatoma and otorrhea does not result in cessation of suppuration caused by sequestration and loculation of disease within the mastoid cell system.

Access to the sinus tympani

The sinus tympani is notorious for harboring residual disease, either cholesteatoma, granulation, or both, and for difficulty in accessing it. Access to the sinus tympani can be facilitated significantly by first identifying the vertical segment of the facial nerve, and then removing the triangle of bone between the vertical segment of the nerve and the middle ear space, which overlies sinus tympani (Fig. 10). Such modification also significantly facilitates access to the hypotympanic cell system, if needed.

Modifications to prevent recurrence

Meatoplasty

In both canal wall up and canal wall down procedures, an adequate meatoplasty, facilitated by removing a crescent of conchal cartilage from the posterior aspect of the ear canal (Fig. 11), greatly facilitates postoperative aural hygiene and inspection.

Canalplasty

Canalplasty (particularly in a tortuous or narrow ear canal), accomplished by removing bone from the tympanic segment of the external auditory canal, greatly facilitates access, both intraoperatively and postoperatively. Widening and straightening the canal also helps to prevent

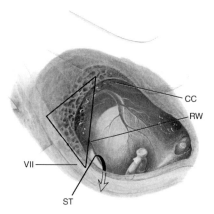

Fig. 10. Access to the sinus tympani (ST), which is located medial to the facial nerve (VII) and to the hypotympanic cells, is facilitated by removal of bone between the facial nerve (VII), round window (RW), and carotid canal (CC), as shown in the triangle. (*From* Nadol JB, McKenna MJ. Surgery of the ear and temporal bone. 2nd edition. Philadelphia: Lippincott, Williams and Wilkins; 2005; with permission.)

postoperative stenosis, particularly at the anterior angle between the tympanic membrane and the somewhat oblique anterior canal wall (Fig. 12).

Graft stiffening procedures

Recurrent disease for both canal wall up and canal wall down procedures is often preceded by retraction of the tympanic membrane, particularly in an ear with residual poor tubal function. In an effort to prevent this, stiffening procedures, including use of cartilage grafts either from the tragus or more posterior auricle, as underlay or palisading grafts, helps prevent such retraction.

Exteriorization of cholesteatoma that cannot be removed easily or reliably

Although cholesteatoma generally does not adhere to the facial nerve, it may well adhere to exposed dura of either the middle or posterior cranial fossa. In such cases, obliteration of questionable areas should not be done; such areas should be exteriorized.

In the case of dehiscence of the semicircular canals, careful dissection is often rewarded with clean separation of the cholesteatoma matrix from the underlying endosteum of the vestibular labyrinth. However, when there is a cochlear dehiscence, such an attempt is likely to result in creation of a fistula and significant sensorineural hearing loss. In such cases, with cholesteatomatous cochlear dehiscence, or even dehiscences of the vestibular system in an only hearing or better hearing ear, a staged removal of the entire cholesteatoma is advisable. Thus, removal of the bulk of the cholesteatoma

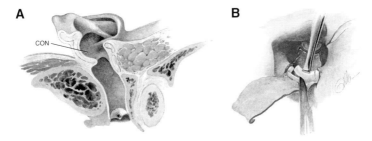

Fig. 11. Meatoplasty. (*A*) The normal meatus is limited posteriorly by overhanging cartilage of the concha (CON). (*B*) A crescent of this cartilage may be removed to enlarge the natural meatus. (*From* Nadol JB, McKenna MJ. Surgery of the ear and temporal bone. 2nd edition. Philadelphia: Lippincott, Williams and Wilkins; 2005; with permission.)

from the site, while leaving the cholesteatomatous epithelium intact, allows osseous healing beneath it over the passage of months, and facilitates a second-look completion procedure.

Indications for obliterative techniques for canal wall down revision tympanomastoidectomy

Indications for obliteration of the mastoid include a desire to minimize the cavity size and to provide a stable, viable, soft-tissue barrier between overlying skin and bone and critical structures, such as the labyrinth and facial nerve. This eliminates or greatly decreases the difficulty in postoperative aural hygiene of the mastoid bowl; reduces the incidence of recurrent retraction; and helps prevent remucosalization of unexenerated cells, particularly in the mastoid tip, sinodural angle, and tegmental areas.

In a chronic ear with no residual cochlear function, total tympanomastoidectomy significantly reduces the postoperative healing time and required postoperative maintenance, but is contingent upon confidence in the total removal of disease and in the ability to clinically follow such patients over time, both in the office and, if necessary, with postoperative imaging.

Techniques for obliteration of the canal wall down mastoid bowl

After a complete exenteration of disease and residual cells with granulation, an often overlooked technique that results in reduction of the size of the bowl is to eliminate the lateral bony portion of the mastoid tip to the level of the digastric muscle. Additional modalities include the use of musculoperiosteal flaps, either superiorly or inferiorly based; fibroperiosteal flaps with temporalis extension or with subtemporalis periosteal extension [22]; wing flaps, as advocated by Bruce Black [23]; and the use of bone pate (Fig. 13) [24]. Total tympanomastoid obliteration can be achieved with abdominal fat, with or without adjunctive materials such as musculoperiosteal or fibroperiosteal flaps, or with vascularized rotational flaps such as the temporoparietal fascial flap [25].

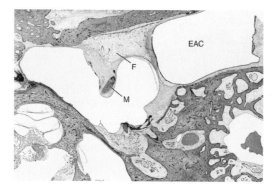

Fig. 12. Blunting of the external auditory canal. The space between the manubrium (M) and the anterior wall of the external auditory canal (EAC) has been filled with fibrous tissue (F).

Split thickness skin grafting

Although split thickness skin grafting may be delayed until the postoperative period, it is the author's preference, particularly in revision tympanomastoidectomy, to incorporate intraoperative split thickness skin grafting from the upper arm to critical areas such as the anterior canal wall, in an effort to control postoperative fibrosis and stenosis. Although an avascular temporalis fascial graft will not have sufficient blood supply for several weeks to accept the split thickness skin graft, the placement of adjacent grafts on the anterior and inferior canal wall may preclude the need for such subsequent grafting. In contrast, a well-vascularized rotational flap, such as the temporoparietal fascial flap, will accept immediate split thickness skin grafting.

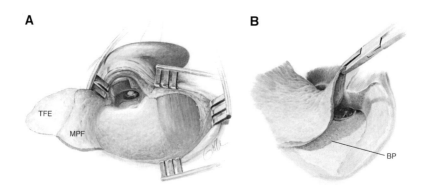

Fig. 13. Obliteration of the mastoid bowl. (*A*) In this left ear, a musculoperiosteal flap (MPF) with an extension of temporalis fascia (TFE) has been elevated, based on the mastoid tip. (*B*) This flap is used later to cover bone pate (BP) placed in the exenterated canal wall down mastoid bowl. (*From* Nadol JB, McKenna MJ. Surgery of the ear and temporal bone. 2nd edition. Philadelphia: Lippincott, Williams and Wilkins; 2005; with permission.)

The use of alloplastic stenting material

Although placement of allograft material in the middle ear may result occasionally in a foreign body reaction, silastic sheeting may be very helpful to prevent stenosis and adhesion between graft material, such as temporalis fascia, and a significantly damaged middle ear mucosa. The aeration of the mastoid in a canal wall up procedure may also be maintained by placing a silastic sheet between the middle ear space and the central mastoid tract, by way of the facial recess.

Summary

Achieving a safe, dry ear over the long term in chronic active otitis media with or without cholesteatoma often requires revision surgery; initial failure rates approach 30% of cases in some series. Categorizing and locating the recurrent disease process, and analyzing the reasons for previous failure, are necessary to plan a successful revision surgical procedure. It is also necessary to be aware of the various histopathologic correlates of chronic otitis media, including osteoresorptive and osteosclerotic processes. In addition to complete removal of disease, modifications to prevent recurrent disease, including meatoplasty, canalplasty, graft stiffening procedures, and obliterative techniques, may be used. Careful attention to detail and analysis of the reasons for previous surgical failure will lead to a customized, case-specific plan that may require modification during the course of the procedure, based on surgical findings.

References

[1] Jepsen O, Swergius E. Cavities after retro-auricular radical ear operations with special reference to significance of primary factors. Acta Otolaryngol 1951;39:388–94.

[2] Ohrt HH. On recurrence in cavities after radical mastoidectomy with special reference to the complications which may arise. Acta Otolaryngol (Stockh.) 1957;47:346–52.

[3] Smyth GD. Postoperative cholesteatoma in combined approach tympanoplasty. J Laryngol Otol 1976;90:597–621.

[4] Sheehy J, Brackmann DE, Graham MD. Cholesteatoma surgery: residual and recurrent disease. A review of 1,024 cases. Ann Otol 1977;86:451–62.

[5] Palmgren O. Long term results of open cavity and tympanomastoid surgery of the chronic ear. Acta Otolaryngol 1979;88(5–6):343–9.

[6] Van Baarle PW, Juygen PL, Brinkman WF. Findings in surgery for chronic otitis media. A retrospective data-analysis of 2225 cases followed for 2 years. Clin Otolaryngol Allied Sci 1983;8(3):151–8.

[7] Cody DTR, McDonald TJ. Mastoidectomy for acquired cholesteatoma: follow-up to 20 years. Laryngoscope 1984;94:1027–30.

[8] Lau T, Tos M. Long term results of surgery for chronic granulating otitis. Am J Otolaryngol 1986;7(5):341–5.

[9] Pillsbury HC 3rd, Carrasco VN. Revision mastoidectomy. Arch Otolaryngol Head Neck Surg 1990;116(9):1019–22.

[10] Vartiainen E, Kansanen M. Tympanomastoidectomy for chronic otitis media without cholesteatoma. Otolaryngol Head Neck Surg 1992;106(3):230–4.

[11] Syms MJ, Luxford WM. Management of cholesteatoma: status of the canal wall. Laryngoscope 2003;113(3):443–8.

[12] Kos MI, Castrillon R, Montandon P, et al. Anatomic and functional long term results of canal wall-down mastoidectomy. Ann Otol Rhinol Laryngol 2004;113(11):872–6.

[13] Merchant SN, Wang P, Jang CH, et al. Efficacy of tympanomastoid surgery for control of
infection in active chronic otitis media. Laryngoscope 1997;107(7):872–7.

[14] Richardson GS. Aditus block. Ann Otol Rhinol Laryngol 1963;72:223–36.

[15] Proctor B. Attic-aditus block and the tympanic diaphragm. Ann Otol Rhinol Laryngol 1971;
80(3):371–5.

[16] Jokippi AM, Karma P, Ojala K, et al. Anaerobic bacteria in chronic otitis media. Arch Otolaryngol 1977;103(5):278–80.

[17] Erkan M, Aslan T, Sevuk E, et al. Bacteriology of chronic suppurative otitis media. Ann Otol
Rhinol Laryngol 1994;103:771–4.

[18] Kenna M, Bluestone CD, Reilly JS, et al. Medical management of chronic suppurative otitis
media without cholesteatoma in children. Laryngoscope 1986;96:146–51.

[19] Nadol JB Jr. Causes of failure of mastoidectomy for chronic otitis media. Laryngoscope
1985;95(4):410–3.

[20] Nadol JB Jr, Krouse JH. The hypotympanum and infralabyrinthine cells in chronic otitis
media. Laryngoscope 1991;101:137–41.

[21] Rambo JHJ. The use of musculoplasty: Advantages and disadvantages. Ann Otol 1965;74:
535–54.

[22] Ramsey MJ, Merchant SN, McKenna MJ. Postauricular periosteal-pericranial flap for mastoid obliteration and canal wall down tympanomastoidectomy. Otol Neurotol 2004;25(6):
873–8.

[23] Black B. Mastoidectomy elimination: obliterate, reconstruct, or ablate? Am J Otol 1998;
19(5):551–7.

[24] Sheehy JL. Bone pate collecting device. Otolaryngol Head Neck Surg 1980;88(4):472.

[25] Cheney ML, Megerian CA, Brown MT, et al. The use of the temporoparietal fascial flap in
temporal bone reconstruction. Am J Otol 1996;17:137–42.

ELSEVIER
SAUNDERS

Otolaryngol Clin N Am
39 (2006) 741–750

OTOLARYNGOLOGIC
CLINICS
OF NORTH AMERICA

Revision Surgery for Vertigo

John F. Kveton, MD*

*Department of Surgery/Otolaryngology, Yale University School of Medicine,
New Haven, CT*

Vertigo after otologic surgery can be either a complication of a particular procedure or a failure of a procedure designed to eradicate the symptom of vertigo. These situations are substantially different because the cause of the symptom of vertigo is so dissimilar. Despite the different causes of the symptoms, the reality is that the ultimate choice of procedure to control the vertigo may be the same. Our discussion of the management of vertigo after otologic procedures focuses on the origin of the vertigo rather than the procedure required to eradicate the symptom.

Vertigo after stapedectomy

The development of vertigo after stapedectomy or stapedotomy is not uncommon in the immediate postoperative period. Vertigo may be spontaneous in the immediate postoperative period but is more commonly associated with positional changes. Positional vertigo rarely lasts longer than several days to 1 week after surgery and demonstrates slow improvement over time. The development of worsening vertigo, usually episodic but at times positionally induced, should alert a surgeon that surgical intervention may be necessary. Sensorineural hearing loss simultaneous with vertigo makes this an urgent surgical situation. Severe to profound hearing loss associated with vertigo is a surgical emergency. Fluctuating hearing loss with associated auditory symptoms, such as tinnitus and aural fullness, can be assessed in a more leisurely fashion. The configuration of the audiogram may be helpful in determining whether surgical intervention is necessary. A low-frequency sensorineural hearing loss most likely indicates that a patient has developed Meniere's syndrome, for which re-exploration of the oval window region proves fruitless to reduce symptoms. A flat, severe to

* 46 Prince Street, Suite 601, New Haven, CT 06519-1634.
E-mail address: john.kveton@yale.edu

0030-6665/06/$ - see front matter © 2006 Elsevier Inc. All rights reserved.
doi:10.1016/j.otc.2006.03.002   *oto.theclinics.com*

profound sensorineural hearing loss or a severe to profound high-frequency sensorineural hearing loss, especially with reduced speech discrimination, requires immediate surgical attention.

Perilymphatic fistula is the foremost cause for vertigo (and hearing loss) after stapedectomy (total footplate removal). Migration of the tissue seal is the most likely cause if vertigo persists through the perioperative period, and immediate surgical intervention is necessary to prevent permanent hearing loss or vertigo. When not occurring in the immediate postoperative period, perilymphatic fistula is usually produced by precipitating factors, such as barotrauma (especially associated with an acute sinusitis or severe upper respiratory tract illness), sudden increase in intracranial pressure, or head trauma that tears or displaces the tissue seal in the oval window. In cases in which a stapedotomy has been performed, these events cause a displacement of the prosthesis out of the stapedotomy hole with resultant perilymphatic fluid leak.

The surgical repair of the perilymphatic fistula requires a revision stapedectomy. A new piece of soft tissue (the author prefers perichondrium) should be harvested before the development of the tympanomeatal flap. Once the middle ear is exposed, any adhesions in the vicinity of the oval window niche should be lysed carefully. The stapes prosthesis should be isolated from any adhesions to the tissue seal in the oval window (or to the stapedotomy defect) and removed from the long process of the incus. Using high-power magnification, further adhesions should be removed from the oval window region in proximity to the tissue seal, which can be accomplished with small micropicks or laser vaporization. In cases of a perioperative exploration, replacement of the existing soft tissue seal should be performed. In cases of delayed perilymphatic fistula after stapedectomy, the existing tissue seal should not be removed completely because adhesions may have developed between the macule of the utricle and the tissue seal. Because disruption of such adhesions may lead to deafness, the residual soft tissue should be cleaned of mucosal adhesions as much as possible and the oval window niche should be resurfaced with the new piece of tissue. Revision surgery in a previous stapedotomy is best managed by removal of at least one half of the footplate and placement of a generous piece of soft tissue to cover the oval window. Remeasurement for prosthesis length should be attempted before footplate removal, especially if the original surgeon is not performing the revision procedure. Too deep a placement of the initial prosthesis should be recognizable at the time of surgery, but this situation is usually determined by a temporal bone CT scan before revision surgery.

The delayed appearance of vertigo after stapedectomy may be associated with the development of Meniere's syndrome in a small number of patients. The coexistence of otosclerosis and Meniere's disease has been recognized for many years, and a preoperative history of vertigo should alert the surgeon to the possibility of this disorder [1,2]. The induction of Meniere's syndrome after stapedectomy is rarer, but this condition must be differentiated from perilymphatic fistula because the vertigo associated with Meniere's syndrome is not cured by surgical exploration. Fortunately, this differential diagnosis usually can be made through analysis of the audiogram. As in most patients who have Meniere's disease, low-frequency sensorineural hearing loss is the predominant feature observed on the audiogram, which is in contrast to the high-frequency sensorineural hearing loss observed in most cases of perilymphatic fistula. As in most cases of early Meniere's disease, speech discrimination scores are usually good in cases of Meniere's syndrome after stapedectomy, whereas speech discrimination scores tend to deteriorate more rapidly in cases of a perilymphatic fistula. Medical management of this condition with diuretic therapy and low sodium diet should be instituted immediately.

If vertigo persists after revision stapedectomy, the options for vertigo control revolve around the residual hearing present after the revision procedure. In most cases of persistent vertigo, hearing loss is significant and is a reflection of the damage that has occurred in the inner ear. Once the vestibular damage has been confirmed to be peripheral (and central disorders ruled out) by vestibular testing, labyrinthectomy should be recommended to eliminate the vertigo. Although it is tempting to consider the transcanal approach, a transmastoid labyrinthectomy should be performed to ensure that all neuroepithelium (especially the posterior canal ampulla) is removed. In rare cases in which vertigo persists in the presence of serviceable hearing (<50 dB speech reception threshold, >50% speech discrimination score), vestibular neurectomy can be considered. In no case should intratympanic gentamicin be considered to ablate vestibular function. Intratympanic therapy is indicated in the management of Meniere's disease in patients who have not had previous middle ear procedures.

Vertigo after surgery for Meniere's disease

The persistence of vertigo after procedures to control these symptoms of Meniere's disease is highly variable and depends on the type of the initial procedure used. The most effective procedure to control vertigo associated with Meniere's disease is the transmastoid labyrinthectomy [3]. The results of transcanal labyrinthectomy are comparable in experienced hands, and these two surgical procedures are more effective than chemical labyrinthectomy procedures. Vestibular neurectomy carries a success rate of vertigo control of more than 90% [4,5]. It has greater possible morbidity than surgical labyrinthectomy but also has the advantage of hearing preservation in most cases. Chemical labyrinthectomy has a lower rate of vertigo elimination [6,7] and has a rate of recurrent vertigo that ranks it close to endolymphatic sac surgery in terms of failure to control the vertigo symptoms associated with Meniere's disease [8–10]. The remainder of this article outlines an approach to the surgical decision making in regards to managing recurrent vertigo after these procedures.

Vertigo after chemical labyrinthectomy

Although the least invasive of all procedures to control vertigo in Meniere's disease, chemical labyrinthectomy carries a higher risk of sensorineural hearing loss than endolymphatic sac procedures while providing a higher rate of vertigo control. Although the incidence of hearing complications may be dose dependent, the incidence of recurrent vertigo also seems to be associated with single or limited dosing [5,11]. Vertigo control rates range from 80% to 90%, but there is no differentiation between persistent vertigo and recurrence of vertigo after what was considered a successful procedure [12,13]. The management of these two groups of patients (ie, persistent versus delayed vertigo) varies depending on several variables, including hearing loss, extent of vestibular function, and the time period since last injection.

Successful chemical labyrinthectomy occurs if a patient experiences a severe vertigo attack followed by disequilibrium that lasts for weeks to months after an injection. Depending on the surgeon, patients undergo one to three injections of gentamicin to achieve this result. If vertigo recurs weeks after the initial postinjection vertigo, the patient should be considered a failure to this procedure, and alternative methods of controlling vertigo should be entertained. Caloric testing and audiometric testing must be performed to determine whether vestibular function persists in the gentamicin-exposed ear and to confirm auditory status. The choice of a destructive or conservative surgical procedure in such a situation depends on the auditory reserve at that time.

The reappearance of vertigo months to years after chemical labyrinthectomy requires the same audiometric and vestibular evaluation to determine whether unilateral or bilateral Meniere's disease exists. Once the persistence of vestibular function in the chemical labyrinthectomized ear is confirmed with ice water caloric testing, the choice of treatment depends on the auditory reserve identified by audiometric testing. The presence of nonserviceable hearing (>50 dB, <50% speech discrimination score) calls for a destructive procedure to eliminate vertigo definitively. Some authors may advocate for repeat intratympanic gentamicin injections, and there is no doubt that this approach is the least invasive and carries a lower potential morbidity than general anesthesia necessary to perform a transmastoid labyrinthectomy. Such an approach should be entertained in elderly or medically infirm patients who may be at a high risk for the associated morbidity of general anesthesia. Repeat chemical labyrinthectomy can be performed regardless of auditory reserve, and in most instances, the hearing is of minor concern. The number of injections necessary to eliminate vestibular function varies and can be confirmed only by ice water caloric testing. It should be remembered that vestibular function can reappear months later after loss of caloric function because of the toxic effect of gentamicin on vestibular hair cells in the immediate treatment period, not actual cell death. Once energy stores have been replenished to the hair cells, some recovery of hair cell function is possible, with return of symptoms [14].

Because of the inability to predict total vestibular hair cell destruction with chemical labyrinthectomy, there is no argument that surgical labyrinthectomy—in particular transmastoid labyrinthectomy—is the most effective method to eliminate vestibular function. In cases of recurrent vertigo in the presence of nonserviceable hearing after chemical labyrinthectomy, transmastoid labyrinthectomy should be the first choice in a patient who is medically stable to undergo a general anesthesia. This procedure is particularly effective in cases of progressive Meniere's disease that can be recognized by hearing deterioration since the chemical labyrinthectomy. In such cases, because auditory reserve is no longer a concern, the rapid elimination of vestibular function via surgery allows a patient to return to normal function in a more timely, organized fashion than waiting for the gentamicin to take effect after the injections. An added benefit of transmastoid labyrinthectomy compared with chemical labyrinthectomy is the lower incidence of disequilibrium associated with surgical labyrinthectomy. Persistent imbalance is more common in chemical labyrinthectomy and can be as debilitating as vertigo. These symptoms are improved after surgical removal of all neuroepithelium.

The presence of serviceable hearing with persistent vertigo after chemical labyrinthectomy presents a more complicated dilemma. The two surgical options for vertigo control in the presence of serviceable hearing in Meniere's disease are endolymphatic sac surgery and vestibular neurectomy. It is tempting to consider endolymphatic sac surgery as the first option in cases of persistent vertigo after chemical ablation because it is the less invasive of the two procedures. A brief review of the timing of the use of endolymphatic sac surgery in the management of patients with Meniere's disease would reveal that this procedure should have limited use in revision surgery after chemical labyrinthectomy. Endolymphatic sac surgery is the least effective, although the least invasive, procedure to control vertigo in Meniere's disease. The procedure is considered the first-line surgical procedure when hearing is serviceable and vestibular function is still present, because the aim of the procedure is to alter the hydropic state in the inner ear to preserve hearing and vestibular function. If a chemical labyrinthectomy has been performed (whose purpose is to destroy vestibular function), the likelihood of further damage to the vestibular system is high, and the metabolic state of the inner ear may be affected permanently. In this situation, even in the presence of serviceable hearing, this additional damage puts a patient's inner ear into a later stage of Meniere's disease and so it is less likely to respond to endolymphatic sac manipulation. Endolymphatic sac surgery should be considered only as a revision surgical option in cases of serviceable hearing with evidence of no or minimal damage to the vestibular system on caloric testing.

Because caloric testing almost always reveals vestibular damage after chemical ablation, the only surgical procedure to consider in the presence of serviceable hearing is vestibular neurectomy. Repeated gentamicin injection is another option, but because the potential for hearing loss increases with dosage, the safest means to eliminate vertigo is to perform a vestibular neurectomy.

Vertigo after endolymphatic sac surgery

Recurrent vertigo after endolymphatic sac surgery statistically occurs more commonly than any other procedure performed to control vertigo in Meniere's disease. Endolymphatic sac surgery is the most conservative surgical procedure, and it has the express purpose of changing the endolymphatic environment, not destroying vestibular function. The effect of endolymphatic sac surgery does not result in one last severe episode of vertigo followed by 6 to 8 weeks of vestibular compensation. Rather it results in a reduction and hopeful elimination of the severity and frequency of the vertigo attacks. There is no definitive time frame that determines when success should be measured after endolymphatic sac surgery, because no scientific data have documented how endolymphatic sac surgery affects the endolymphatic system. It is up to the surgeon to determine the period of time to consider this procedure a failure in controlling vertigo. Determination of failure can be relative rather than absolute, depending on the frequency and severity of vertigo and the effect that vertigo attacks have on a patient's daily activities. Barring the persistence of weekly disabling attacks of vertigo, aggressive medical management with diuretics and vestibular suppressants should continue for at least 3 months after endolymphatic sac surgery until the procedure has been deemed a failure. If vertigo attacks persistent but are less frequent and severe, perseverance with the medical management should be recommended as long as progress is being demonstrated.

Once endolymphatic sac surgery has been deemed unsuccessful, the choice of revision procedure depends on the auditory and vestibular status after the endolymphatic sac surgery. If serviceable hearing remains, regardless of vestibular function, a hearing preservation procedure should be performed. If vestibular function is normal or shows minimal damage, one may be tempted to consider a revision endolymphatic sac procedure. Few data support the effectiveness of this procedure, and the author's personal bias is not to consider performing a revision endolymphatic sac procedure if one is sure that the endolymphatic sac has been decompressed widely at the initial procedure.

Regardless of the degree of vestibular function, the existence of recurrent vertigo and serviceable hearing after endolymphatic sac surgery leads to consideration of either chemical labyrinthectomy or vestibular neurectomy as a means to ablate vestibular function. The effectiveness of chemical labyrinthectomy to control vertigo after endolymphatic sac surgery is debatable. Although it is an attractive alternative to the more invasive and potentially morbid neurectomy, vertigo control rates in such cases are lower than in initial cases [15]. Such lower control rates have been hypothesized to occur because of the migration of bone particles during drilling into the round window niche. The more effective method to control vertigo in these cases is vestibular neurectomy. Surgical exposure to the vestibular nerve is not compromised by the previous endolymphatic sac procedure, with ready identification of the vestibular nerve, and causes no greater complication rate compared with vestibular neurectomy as the primary procedure for control of vertigo in Meniere's disease.

When vertigo persists in the presence of nonserviceable hearing after endolymphatic sac surgery, transmastoid labyrinthectomy should be performed unless a patient is medically unfit for general anesthesia. Although chemical labyrinthectomy can be attempted with no limit to the number of injections because hearing is not an issue, the rapidity and assured result obtained by surgical labyrinthectomy in a patient who already has opted for surgical methods to control vertigo seems the most logical choice. The surgeon must keep in mind the psychological and economic impact that vertigo has on a patient and that a definitive procedure such as a surgical labyrinthectomy, with a known starting point for recovery, goes a long way in aiding recovery.

Vertigo after vestibular neurectomy

The recurrence of vertigo after vestibular neurectomy is unusual, occurring in less than 10% of patients, and is attributed to incomplete sectioning of the vestibular nerve. This condition can be documented readily by ice water caloric testing. Auditory status at the time of recurrent symptoms dictates the approach that should be used to eliminate vertigo. In the presence of serviceable hearing, a revision neurectomy is the most effective means to control the symptoms. The selection of the approach for the neurectomy may be a factor in such cases. Lower success rates of vestibular neurectomy have been noted in retrosigmoid or suboccipital neurectomies compared with middle fossa neurectomy [16]. In these procedures the vestibular nerve is usually sectioned in the cerebellopontine angle by noting the cleavage plane between the auditory nerve and the vestibular nerve trunks as the VIIIth nerve exits the brainstem. Especially in cases in which the cleavage plane is indistinct, there is a chance that some vestibular nerve fibers may be left behind, resulting in an incomplete neurectomy. Theoretically, identifying the vestibular nerve distal to this region (ie, within the internal auditory canal) should reduce the possibility of incomplete neurectomy. This assurance can be accomplished by drilling the internal auditory canal posteriorly (via suboccipital or retrosigmoid approaches) or superiorly (via a middle cranial fossa approach). Some authors insist that the more distal the better, so that identification of the vestibular nerves as they enter the bony labyrinth affords the best results. This type of neurectomy can be performed only via the middle cranial fossa approach, which also would also provide a better chance of severing any vestibulocochlear anastamoses, which may have some effect on recurrent symptoms after what was thought to be a complete neurectomy. The concern in this situation is whether any increase in morbidity that may be associated with a neurectomy at the fundus of the internal auditory canal is worth the risk. Exposure of the fundus of the internal auditory canal requires exposure of the labyrinthine segment of the facial nerve and the basal turn of the cochlea, which increases the risk of deafness and facial paralysis in this procedure. Although the published data show little difference in complication rates, it is the author's opinion that such a revision procedure should be performed only by a surgeon who is well versed in the middle cranial fossa anatomy.

The recurrence of vertigo after vestibular neurectomy associated with nonserviceable hearing can be controlled readily by transmastoid labyrinthectomy. This procedure carries lower potential morbidity for a patient than a revision neurectomy and is better tolerated. The recovery time necessary after this procedure is usually less than after the initial neurectomy because most vestibular function already has been ablated. It is not unusual for such patients to leave the hospital on the first postoperative day with minimal imbalance, unlike the severe imbalance noted after the initial procedure.

In cases of recurrent vertigo after vestibular neurectomy, regardless of auditory status, it is tempting to consider chemical labyrinthectomy as an alternative to surgical ablation. The unpredictability of this procedure, despite the fact that it is the least invasive, makes it a less attractive option unless intervening medical issues make surgical intervention unacceptable. When serviceable hearing is present, the risk of hearing loss is higher than in revision neurectomy, whereas the presence of reduced vestibular function in no way suggests that only one course of gentamicin is successful to eliminate the persistent vestibular function. Especially in cases of nonserviceable hearing, a surgeon can eliminate vertigo via surgical labyrinthectomy, thereby ensuring that a patient will be able to resume normal activities in a timely manner. Such definitive assurances cannot be made when performing chemical labyrinthectomy.

Vertigo after surgical labyrinthectomy

The recurrence of vertigo after surgical labyrinthectomy is rare. Transcanal labyrinthectomy has been associated with a higher rate of recurrence because of the lack of visualization of the posterior canal ampulla at the time of the procedure. Transmastoid labyrinthectomy eliminates this potential cause for failure of surgical labyrinthectomy. Recurrence of vertigo after transmastoid labyrinthectomy should raise concern for several conditions. If symptoms recur years after the initial procedure, reimaging with MRI should be performed to rule out an intracranial process. Ice water caloric testing and audiometric testing should be performed. In almost every case of recurrent vertigo after transmastoid labyrinthectomy, contralateral Meniere's disease is identified, and the normal treatment protocol for unilateral Meniere's disease should be instituted. In the unlikely event that vestibular function persists in the operated ear, a revision transmastoid labyrinthectomy should be performed with VIIIth nerve section. If caloric function is absent in the operated ear and all audiometric testing is normal in the contralateral ear, other causes of vertigo must be considered. The most prominent possibility is vertigo associated with migraine disorder, and a neurologic consultation should be made.

Vertigo after repair of spontaneous perilymphatic fistula

Intraoperative identification and surgical repair of a spontaneous perilymphatic fistula carries a high rate of success for vertigo control. Persistence of vertigo after the procedure requires a different approach than recurrence of vertigo some time after a successful procedure. After successful repair of a perilymphatic fistula, vertigo symptoms disappear quickly. If vertigo symptoms are unchanged weeks after the procedure, additional procedures are necessary to control the symptoms if medical management is not successful. The choice of the procedure, as in previous discussions, depends primarily on the auditory reserve after the initial procedure. In the presence of serviceable hearing, vestibular neurectomy is the treatment of choice. Transmastoid labyrinthectomy should be performed when vertigo persists with nonserviceable hearing.

When vertigo recurs after successful closure of a perilymphatic fistula, the options for surgical repair can be less extreme, depending on audiometric status at the time of recurrent symptoms. Most often perilymphatic fistula is associated with a high-frequency sensorineural hearing loss, with reduced speech discrimination. If the audiogram demonstrates low-frequency sensorineural hearing loss, the development of endolymphatic hydrops should be suspected. The usual medical treatment that involves diuretics and low sodium diet should be instituted. If pre-existing high-frequency sensorineural hearing loss remains stable or deteriorates, a revision perilymphatic fistula repair can be considered. This approach is the most conservative means to control the recurrence. Once the surgical site has been re-exposed, the tissue seal in the oval or round window should be removed completely and replaced with perichondrium after all mucosa surrounding the window has been removed.

Because the success of a revision fistula repair is variable, more effective procedures to control vertigo would involve vestibular ablative procedures, such as vestibular neurectomy or transmastoid labyrinthectomy. The selection of these procedures depends on auditory status at the time of symptoms.

Summary

The management of recurrent vertigo after otologic procedures requires a disciplined approach to evaluate auditory and vestibular reserve before embarking on a revision procedure. Knowledge of the underlying disorder that prompted the initial procedure, coupled with an understanding of the pathophysiology involved in the persistence or recurrence of the vertigo, allows a surgeon to choose an appropriate procedure to eradicate vertigo with minimum attendant morbidity for the patient.

References

[1] Sismanis A, Hughes GB, Abedi E. Coexisting otosclerosis and Meniere's disease: a diagnostic and therapeutic dilemma. Laryngoscope 1986;96:9–13.

[2] Paparella MM, Mancini I, Liston SL. Otosclerosis and Meniere's syndrome: diagnosis and treatment. Laryngoscope 1984;94:1414–7.

[3] Gacek RR, Gacek MR. Comparison of labyrinthectomy and vestibular neurectomy in the control of vertigo. Laryngoscope 1996;106:225–30.

[4] Tewary AK, Riley N, Kerr AG. Long-term results of vestibular nerve section. J Laryngol Otol 1998;112:1150–3.

[5] Pappas DG Jr, Pappas DG Sr. Vestibular nerve section: long-term follow-up. Laryngoscope 1997;107:1203–9.

[6] Hillman TA, Chen DA, Arriaga MA. Vestibular nerve section versus intratympanic gentamicin for Meniere's disease. Laryngoscope 2004;114:216–22.

[7] Chia SH, Gamst AC, Anderson JP, et al. Intratympanic gentamicin therapy for Meniere's disease: a meta-analysis. Otol Neurotol 2005;25:544–52.

[8] Harner SG, Driscoll CL, Facer GW, et al. Long-term follow-up of transtympanic gentamicin for Meniere's syndrome. Otol Neurotol 2001;22:210–4.

[9] Ostrowski VB, Kartush JM. Endolymphatic sac-vein decompression for intractable Meniere's disease: long term treatment results. Otolaryngol Head Neck Surg 2003;128:550–9.

[10] Pensak ML, Friedman RA. The role of endolymphatic mastoid shunt surgery in the managed care era. Am J Otol 1998;19:337–40.

[11] Light JP, Silverstein H, Jackson LE. Gentamicin perfusion vestibular response and hearing loss. Otol Neurotol 2003;24:294–8.

[12] Kaplan DM, Nedzelski JM, Chen JM, et al. Intratympamic gentamicin for the treatment of unilateral Meniere's disease. Laryngoscope 2000;110:1298–305.

[13] Atlas J, Parnes LS. Intratympamic gentamicin for intractable Meniere's disease: a 5 year follow-up. J Otolaryngol 2003;32:288–93.

[14] Okuda T, Sugahara K, Shimogori H, et al. Inner ear changes with intracochlear gentamicin administration in guinea pigs. Laryngoscope 2004;114:694–7.

[15] Minor LB. Intratympamic gentamicin for control of vertigo in Meniere's disease: vestibular signs that specify completion of therapy. Am J Otol 1999;20:209–19.

[16] Green JD Jr, Shelton C, Brackmann DE. Middle fossa vestibular neurectomy in retrolabyrinthine neurectomy failures. Arch Otolaryngol Head Neck Surg 1992;118:1058–60.

ELSEVIER
SAUNDERS

Otolaryngol Clin N Am
39 (2006) 751–762

OTOLARYNGOLOGIC
CLINICS
OF NORTH AMERICA

Acoustic Neuroma (Vestibular Schwannoma) Revision

Richard J. Wiet, MD, FACS[a,b,c,d,]*,
Robert P. Kazan, MD[b,e], Ivan Ciric, MD[a,f],
Philip D. Littlefield, MD[a]

[a]Northwestern University Feinberg School of Medicine, Chicago, IL, USA
[b]Hinsdale Hospital, Hinsdale, IL, USA
[c]Northwestern Memorial Hospital, Chicago, IL, USA
[d]Ear Institute of Chicago, LLC, Hinsdale, IL, USA
[e]West Suburban Neurosurgical Associates, Hinsdale, IL, USA
[f]Evanston Northwestern Hospital, Evanston, IL, USA

The authors collectively present their experience of more than 25 years, now in excess of 1200 patients, with cerebellopontine angle (CPA) tumors. Of this number, about 850 patients chose operative management, 110 were advised to have management through observation alone, and 30 had stereotactic radiation. The remainder either were lost to follow-up or chose another center or treatment for their care. Two neurosurgeons were primarily involved in the teamwork care of these patients (RK and IC). Details of the first 500 microsurgical resections already appeared in a peer-reviewed paper [1], and the authors look forward to tabulating the 1000th operative case soon.

This article focuses on the management of planned subtotal resection of acoustic tumors in five subjects, and unexpected "residual" discovered by MRI scanning in 10 cases, which represents, to the best of the authors' knowledge, a residual rate of 1% of operated patients. Shelton [2] at the House Clinic reported a similar experience of 0.3% with 5000 translabyrinthine cases. The rate of residual tumor is as high as 19% in some series and in part depends on the surgical approach [3]. As an example, there was an initial planned attempt to preserve hearing in 8 of the authors' 10 patients

* Corresponding author. Ear Institute of Chicago, 950 North York Road, Suite 102, Hinsdale, IL 60521.

E-mail address: r-wiet@northwestern.edu (R.J. Wiet).

who were later identified with residual tumor. The authors have therefore mandated that all patients have postoperative fat-suppressed, gadolinium-enhanced MRI scans, done sequentially over 10 years, to assure that there is no residual tumor. This mandate has been in place since MRI use became common, starting around 1987. For the purpose of this article, the authors did not include their cases of neurofibromatosis (NF2), because these tumors behave differently from unilateral sporadic schwannomas.

Various treatment modalities are available for patients with residual vestibular schwannoma, including repeat scanning to see if the status has changed, stereotactic radiation, or revision surgery. The decision is individualized with the patient, depending on tumor status, preference, and general medical condition. It is beyond the scope of this article to describe how this decision is reached and is referenced in a recent text by one of the authors (RJW) [4].

Materials and methods of follow-up

All patients are told that it is the authors' routine to follow up with scans for 2 years, on the anniversary of the surgery; this practice is discussed during preoperative counseling and in the postoperative period. This cohort is also scanned at 5 and 10 years if no tumor is seen. As a result, four scans over 10 years are required in the postoperative time, if no growth abnormality is seen (Fig. 1). Generally, the postoperative patient who has residual tumor falls into one of two categories: "planned," from near-total or subtotal tumor removal, or "unplanned," discovered by rescanning the patient. These categories are addressed separately.

If there is a suspicion of a tumor or abnormality on the scan, the authors personally review the films with at least two neuroradiologists to confirm suspicion of recurrence. Schmerber and colleagues [5] lay emphasis on cautious interpretation. Surgical manipulation, granulation tissue, and chemical inflammation from blood can create abnormalities that may suggest residual disease. Most of the time, this abnormality is caused by

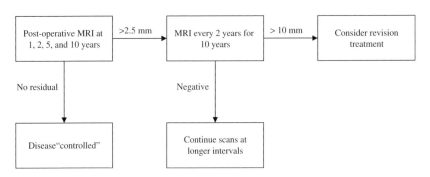

Fig. 1. Postoperative MRI surveillance.

postoperative changes or dural enhancement. Abnormal enhancement occurs in most postoperative MRIs, and serial imaging may be needed to appreciate the significance of an abnormality [6]. MRI scanning may be necessary for life, when suspicion remains.

A database of cases was initiated by one of the authors (RJW), starting in 1980. Currently, this database is being updated for further reporting as one of the larger series of vestibular schwannomas in the authors' region. It involves reviewing the records of every patient with a diagnosis of vestibular schwannoma and entering the information into a Microsoft Access database. The data include gender, age at diagnosis, size and location of tumor, treatment type, cranial nerve function, serial pure-tone averages (PTAs) and speech discrimination, complications, and recurrence. If the patient was treated with surgery, the type of surgery performed is also recorded.

Planned near-total or subtotal resections

As pointed out by Jackler [7], it is prudent to perform less than complete removal of acoustic neuromas, despite the risk of regrowth in certain circumstances, which may mean, for example, leaving a "wafer" of tumor (near-total removal) on the facial nerve to preserve it. This procedure may be planned preoperatively in the elderly. Reoperation is seldom advised if the amount left behind is less than 2 mm. The authors rarely stage surgery, as advocated by Patni and Kartush [8]; however, they aggressively pursue total removal, rather than a planned subtotal removal, in younger patients.

The opposite is true when a large amount of tumor is left after an attempted excision, such as after an adverse turn during surgery. Little is published about these circumstances, but there generally is a higher recurrence rate than with a near-total removal. As an example, the authors have experienced two cases of massive swelling of the cerebellum from venous bleeding that required that the procedure be aborted, despite only partial tumor removal. The authors also terminated two cases with adverse vital sign changes (bradycardia). In these two patients, tumors were in excess of 3.5 cm beyond the porus acusticus, with brainstem indentation. The authors' experience with tumors in this size range has been reported previously [9]. Each subtotal resection resulted in residual tumor much greater than 2.5 mm that was visible on subsequent MRI scans. Three of the four patients chose postoperative Gamma Knife treatment and are stable. One patient (case report #1) required revision surgery, and subsequently a hypoglossal-facial anastomosis for facial reanimation.

Case report #1: subtotal resection

A 52-year-old man presented with hearing loss, tinnitus, and imbalance for one year. The audiogram showed an asymmetric sensorineural hearing loss in the left ear. His PTA was 54 decibels (dB) and his speech discrimination was 64%. An MRI revealed a heterogeneous, intensely enhancing mass in the left CPA and internal auditory canal (IAC) (Fig. 2). The mediolateral measurement was 3.0 cm and cranial-caudal width was nearly 2.0 cm. The tumor was thought initially to be a meningioma because of its peculiar presentation. It grew superiorly toward the geniculate area, instead of having the typical mushroom-like appearance of an acoustic tumor. A planned retrosigmoid operation in August 2004 failed in total

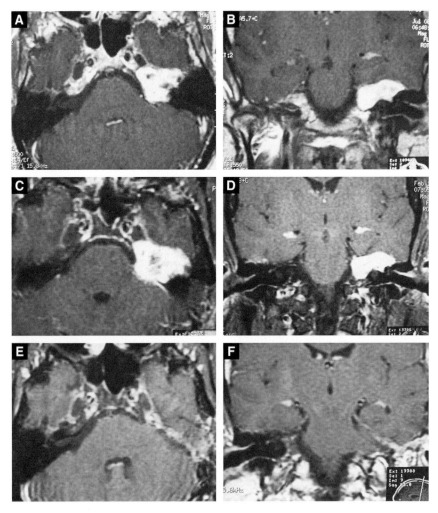

Fig. 2. Subtotal resection (case report #1). (A,B) Preoperative postcontrast T1-weighted MRI (axial and coronal) shows an enhancing left CPA/middle fossa mass. (C,D) Postcontrast T1-weighted MRI with fat suppression (axial and coronal) 6 months after subtotal resection through a retrosigmoid approach. (E,F) Postcontrast T1-weighted MRI (axial with fat suppression, and coronal) 8 months after a transotic revision shows total tumor removal.

removal. A second-stage operation in March 2005 was done from a transotic approach to attack the tumor at the peri-geniculate region. This operation resulted in a facial paralysis that required a hypoglossal-facial anastomosis.

Unplanned residual acoustic tumors

The cases that were discovered by serial scanning with MRI were the result of a 2-decade policy of scanning patients on the anniversary of their surgery, or subsequently. With the exception of 2 out of 10 cases, the tumor was identified the first year. One patient did not adhere to the postoperative instructions and a large tumor was discovered 7 years after a translabyrinthine procedure (case report #2). Surgery for hearing preservation was performed initially in 8 of these 10 cases.

Case report #2: unplanned residual tumor treated with revision surgery

A 49-year-old man initially presented with hearing loss, imbalance, and numbness in the cheek. His facial nerve and lower cranial nerves were otherwise normal. His PTA was 32 dB, with no response to speech discrimination. CT showed a 5-cm right-sided CPA mass that compressed his brainstem about 2.5 cm and caused hydrocephalus. His first surgery was a combined translabyrinthine-suboccipital approach in October 1984. The tumor involved his lower cranial nerves, but they were spared during surgery. He was without symptoms after surgery, but a routine MRI (Fig. 3) in March 1992 showed a recurrent tumor with impingement on the brain stem and cerebellum, medial to the fat graft. It measured 2.5 cm by 1.5 cm. Revision surgery was by the translabyrinthine approach, which was complicated by a facial paralysis that cleared to a House-Brackmann grade III about a year after surgery. Tumor histology confirmed vestibular schwannoma. Proliferation cell division rates of this tumor failed to show anything unusual.

Case report #3: unplanned residual tumor followed by serial MRI

A 50-year-old man presented with right-sided tinnitus of 5 years' duration, and a recently noticed decline in hearing on the same side. An audiogram showed an asymmetric sensorineural hearing loss in the right ear. His PTA was 27 dB and his speech discrimination was 42%. An MRI revealed an enhancing mass that filled the entire right IAC, with 4 mm of extension into the CPA. He had a retrosigmoid resection with hearing preservation in April 1988. The surgeons felt there was complete tumor removal, and the pathology report confirmed vestibular schwannoma. His postoperative PTA was 35 dB, with a speech discrimination of 84%.

The patient was lost initially to follow-up, but returned in September 1993 because of increasing right-sided tinnitus. His hearing was stable,

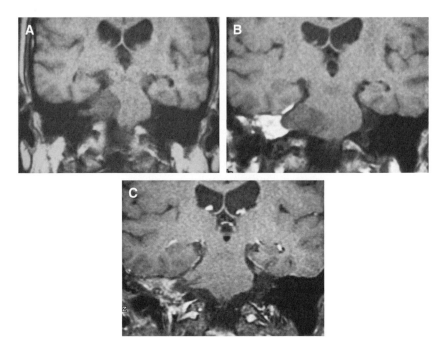

Fig. 3. Unplanned residual tumor (case report #2). (*A*) Preoperative noncontrast T1-weighted MRI in 1984 shows a CPA mass. (*B*) Follow-up noncontrast T1-weighted MRI 7 years later shows residual tumor medial to a fat graft. (*C*) Postcontrast T1-weighted MRI with fat suppression 5 years after translabyrinthine revision does not show tumor.

but an MRI showed an approximately 1.0-cm tumor in the lateral IAC. He has been followed with serial MRI examinations every 2 years since then, and the tumor has not grown. The dimensions as of November 2005 were 10 mm in length, 5 mm in height, and 5 mm in width. His hearing has declined to a PTA of 59 dB, with speech discrimination of 20%. He has normal facial nerve function.

Shelton [2] has illustrated the two likely areas of recurrence of this disease to be remnant tumor not seen in the canal or in the deep recesses of the brain stem. It is possible for schwannoma to be lobulated and hidden from view at the lower cranial nerves, particularly cystic tumors because they tend to compartmentalize. Figure 4 shows two typical areas that may lend themselves to regrowth: near the facial nerve and near the brainstem. Some tumors may develop if not tracked by MRI. Perhaps the most quoted study for understanding the histologic explanation for a recurrence or residual tumor is that of Neely [10]. He demonstrated the microscopic invasion of the seventh and eighth nerves by tumor and questioned the feasibility of total tumor removal with certain hearing preservation techniques. The authors also have had a higher occurrence of tumor residual with this type of case and are in agreement with Yates and colleagues [11], who state that deep

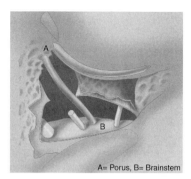

A= Porus, B= Brainstem

Fig. 4. Three likely areas as sources for recurrence: VIIIth nerve stump, facial nerve, and lateral IAC. (*Modified from* Shelton C. Unilateral acoustic tumors: how often do they recur after translabyrinthine removal? Laryngoscope 1995;105(9 Pt 1):958–66.)

involvement of the fundus, with wide erosion of the porus and marginal residual hearing, weigh against the effort of hearing preservation. They argue for a translabyrinthine operation and the authors are in agreement.

The authors have found it expedient to change direction to the translabyrinthine approach when revision surgery is necessary following a retrosigmoid operation. This change gives an excellent, tangential exposure through an unoperated portal. There is minimal cerebellar retraction with small to medium tumors. They recently found it valuable to descend down the tumor capsule, to the cerebellar surface, and to the root-entry zone, which requires careful cerebellar retraction with the Wiet cerebellar retractor or Yasargil flexible system. The authors concentrate on the vestibular-cochlear complex first, and identify the facial nerve about 4 mm medial to that complex. The tumor is debulked progressively, following the seventh-nerve ascent to the petrous ridge, toward the meatus. The neurotologist then identifies the seventh nerve at "Bill's bar" and works the canal component inferiorly toward the brainstem component. This back-and-forth teamwork between the neurotologist and the neurosurgeon pays off immensely in a thorough extirpation of tumor.

Results: near-total resections with follow-up

The authors have tracked patients with near-total removal for 25 years, and the findings have been generally favorable for no growth [1]. Jackler [7] reported a 3% rate of residual in 33 cases, which is similar to what the authors have experienced. Most studies have reported either little or no growth. However, tumor growth 17 years after surgery has been reported [12]. The most common reason for subtotal resection is a concession to hearing preservation in a middle fossa or retrosigmoid operation. The authors try to err on the side of conservatism for the sake of cranial nerve preservation and function. This is possible with tumors as large as 1.0 cm in the IAC during middle fossa surgery, and tumors laterally positioned in the IAC during retrosigmoid removal. To the authors' knowledge, two of the near-total group demonstrated continued slow growth and chose subsequent Gamma Knife radiation.

Results: subtotal resections with follow-up

Results with subtotal resection are not as satisfactory as with total or near-total resection. This finding has been borne out in the literature time and time again [13,14]. The authors have learned to avoid subtotal resections, with two exceptions: the aged patient and for preservation of neurologic function during an adverse turn in surgery.

Generally, if the authors change the surgical direction from retrosigmoid to translabyrinthine, the surgery is fairly straightforward. One must anticipate and carefully dissect through a dense scar plane, which will identify the previously operated region. The hallmark of this is a cerebrospinal fluid (CSF) leak. The tumor is evident following dissection through the scar plane. It will challenge the surgeon to find and preserve the facial nerve. One must adhere to close facial nerve monitoring, because surgical planes and scar distort the usual anatomic landmarks. Stereotactic radiation is an alternative to a second surgical procedure in select cases.

Results: surgery after radiation

The authors have reported previously on tumors that grow after radiation and have found that surgery is more difficult [15]. Fibrosis outside the tumor and within the tumor bed varies and makes the surgery more technically challenging [16]. Light microscopy confirmed the presence of viable tumor cells in all cases of biopsied, radiated tumors. Linthicum [17] also reported this in biopsies of subjects treated with Gamma Knife who required salvage surgery. Additionally, radiation may compromise the patient's ability to respond to an auditory brain stem implant [18].

Facial nerve preservation is less likely with a tumor resection following failed radiosurgery [19–21]. In a recent publication comparing tumor removal between irradiated subjects and a historical control group [21], 46% of the irradiated group had a House-Brackmann grade of 6/6 at the postoperative visit, compared with only 22% of the control group. The facial nerve was severed in 8 of the 38 irradiated cases. The mean diameter of these tumors was 26 mm.

Most centers have lowered their marginal tumor dose from 18 to 20 Gray (Gy), to 13 Gy during the last 15 years [22,23], to decrease the incidence of cranial neuropathies in the fifth, seventh, and eighth nerves. This revised dosing decreased facial neuropathy from 21% to less than 1%, with a 5-year actuarial hearing preservation of 70% [24]. NF2 is much less amenable to radiation treatment. Indeed, as little as 7 months after treatment, young patients with NF2 have shown rapid enlargement of the tumor, suggesting this tumor type is more refractory to radiation [25].

The authors have established some guidelines for radiation avoidance for patients. They are, in order of importance, as follows:

1. Size of the tumor: tumors more than 3 cm in size make tumor control less likely, with the added risk of edema and possible production of hydrocephalus
2. Younger patients under the age of 45 with no surgical risk factors, to eliminate any risk of malignant transformation
3. Patients with cystic, rapidly growing tumors (Fig. 5)
4. Patients with NF2

Discussion

Much discussion in papers on residual and recurrent acoustic tumors focuses on the definitions of how much tumor remains. Shelton [2] has argued for the term "residual" to be used when the surgeon is aware of having left tumor fragments behind. A "recurrent" tumor is thought to be a new tumor that occurs after complete removal of the original tumor; this is an extremely rare event [2]. Sanna [26] has the opinion, based on histologic studies, that the term residual is more appropriate for both conditions.

The problem with most studies, including the authors', is that they are retrospective reviews, and are subject to cases being lost to follow-up. However, an advantage is found in the length of follow-up: 25 years in some instances. Follow-up is the key to detecting residual disease, whether the primary treatment was microsurgery or radiosurgery. Although it is difficult to compare the two types of treatment, the rate of regrowth after treatment appears to be somewhat lower with microsurgery, in series of subjects reported by experienced centers, and can be as low as 0.3% [2]. It is

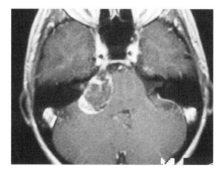

Fig. 5. Rapidly growing cystic tumor. A rapidly growing cystic tumor in a pregnant patient that required surgery during the second trimester. The patient bled into her tumor in the first trimester, prompting the need for intervention.

additionally disconcerting to find proliferation potential in previously radi-ated residual disease [17]. As with microsurgery, the best results are reported in centers with large volumes of experience.

MRI scans are often confusing regarding the significance of postopera-tive findings. Studies by Mueller and colleagues [27] have confirmed that en-hancement around the IAC is common and is to be expected. Indeed, dural enhancement may be present up to 40 years after craniotomy [28]. Postop-erative scar, adhesions, muscle or fat, and trauma to the nerves all must be considered, reinforcing the need for long-term follow-up and MRI protocols after intervention. A unified protocol is needed, but none is in existence as of the date of this writing.

Sanna [26] elucidated symptoms that may suggest a recurrence. These included new facial hypoesthesia and new tinnitus, but they occurred in only 3 of his 23 subjects with recurrences. Because both vestibular and co-chlear symptoms usually are affected by previous treatments, it is necessary to remain vigilant for these changes in status. Most of the authors' patients showed a surprising lack of symptoms, with the exception of those who had late residual greater than 2.5 cm. This finding contrasts with the experiences of Roberson and colleagues [29], who observed symptoms in nearly half of the 33 subjects they evaluated for recurrent tumors.

In many reviews, there appears to be a higher rate of residual after hear-ing preservation surgery, probably because of the canal component of the tumor. The method described by Ciric [30] in a recent article shows how to keep this to a minimum. However, the study by Neely [10] suggests that VIIIth nerve fibers are involved throughout the extent of the tumor, and, in some cases, beyond the tumor's limits, with intraneural invasion by tumor cells. He shows that 500 hertz (Hz) to 2000 Hz audiometry tends to correlate closely with the number of cochlear fibers present, whereas the percentage of unilateral vestibular weakness may not correlate with the fi-bers present in the superior vestibular nerve. The translabyrinthine approach is most appropriate when hearing preservation is unlikely, and it defines more thoroughly the entire length of the tumor, from the IAC to the brainstem. Long-term follow-up with MRI scanning is essential after hearing preserving surgery.

Lastly, there is a newer trend of considering subtotal removal of tumors, followed by postoperative radiation. More long-term studies about this trend are needed. The surgery is essentially a large biopsy in some instances, and is, to the authors, unnecessary, with the single exception being that of a surgery terminated because of life-threatening events.

Summary

Few studies are available today concerning management of residual tu-mor after radiotherapy or microsurgery. Follow-up with serial MRI exam-inations is essential. There appears to be a lower rate of residual tumor with the translabyrinthine operation first described by William House. This approach should be considered in revision cases because it provides excellent exposure of the tumor and surrounding landmarks. Most papers make a plea to create centers of excellence so patients can attain good outcomes. A plea is made herewith to develop a standardized method of postoperative follow-up, no matter how skilled the center believes it is.

References

[1] Wiet RJ, Mamikoglu B, Odom L, et al. Long-term results of the first 500 cases of acoustic neuroma surgery. Otolaryngol Head Neck Surg 2001;124(6):645–51.
[2] Shelton C. Unilateral acoustic tumors: how often do they recur after translabyrinthine removal? Laryngoscope 1995;105(9 Pt 1):958–66.
[3] Cerullo L, Grutsch J, Osterdock R. Recurrence of vestibular (acoustic) schwannomas in surgical patients where preservation of facial and cochlear nerve is the priority. Br J Neurosurg 1998;12(6):547–52.
[4] Wiet RW. Ear and temporal bone surgery: minimizing risks and complications. New York: Thieme Medical Publishers; 2006.
[5] Schmerber S, Palombi O, Boubagra K, et al. Long-term control of vestibular schwannoma after a translabyrinthine complete removal. Neurosurgery 2005;57(4):693–8 [discussion: 8].
[6] Brors D, Schafers M, Bodmer D, et al. Postoperative magnetic resonance imaging findings after transtemporal and translabyrinthine vestibular schwannoma resection. Laryngoscope 2003;113(3):420–6.
[7] Jackler RK, Pfister M. Acoustic neuroma (vestibular schwannoma). In: Jackler RK, Brackmann DE, eds. Neurotology. 2nd edition. Philadelphia: Elsevier Mosby; 2005. p. 727–82.
[8] Patni AH, Kartush JM. Staged resection of large acoustic neuromas. Otolaryngol Head Neck Surg 2005;132(1):11–9.
[9] Mamikoglu B, Wiet RJ, Esquivel CR. Translabyrinthine approach for the management of large and giant vestibular schwannomas. Otol Neurotol 2002;23(2):224–7.
[10] Neely JG. Gross and microscopic anatomy of the eighth cranial nerve in relationship to the solitary schwannoma. Laryngoscope 1981;91(9 Pt 1):1512–31.
[11] Yates PD, Jackler RK, Satar B, et al. Is it worthwhile to attempt hearing preservation in larger acoustic neuromas? Otol Neurotol 2003;24(3):460–4.
[12] Gamache F, Patterson R. Growth rates for residual and recurrent acoustic neuroma. In: Tos M, Thomesn J, eds. Acoustic neuroma. Amsterdam: Kugler; 1992. p. 705–7.
[13] Shea JJ 3rd, Hitselberger WE, Benecke JE Jr, et al. Recurrence rate of partially resected acoustic tumors. Am J Otol 1985;6(Suppl):107–9.
[14] El-Kashlan HK, Zeitoun H, Arts HA, et al. Recurrence of acoustic neuroma after incomplete resection. Am J Otol 2000;21(3):389–92.
[15] Battista RA, Wiet RJ. Stereotactic radiosurgery for acoustic neuromas: a survey of the American Neurotology Society. Am J Otol 2000;21(3):371–81.
[16] Lee DJ, Westra WH, Staecker H, et al. Clinical and histopathologic features of recurrent vestibular schwannoma (acoustic neuroma) after stereotactic radiosurgery. Otol Neurotol 2003;24(4):650–60 [discussion: 60].
[17] Lee F, Linthicum F Jr, Hung G. Proliferation potential in recurrent acoustic schwannoma following gamma knife radiosurgery versus microsurgery. Laryngoscope 2002;112(6):948–50.
[18] Slattery WH 3rd, Brackmann DE. Results of surgery following stereotactic irradiation for acoustic neuromas. Am J Otol 1995;16(3):315–9 [discussion: 9–21].
[19] Pollock BE, Lunsford LD, Kondziolka D, et al. Vestibular schwannoma management. Part II. Failed radiosurgery and the role of delayed microsurgery. J Neurosurg 1998;89(6):949–55.

[20] Roche PH, Regis J, Deveze A, et al. [Surgical removal of unilateral vestibular schwannomas after failed Gamma Knife radiosurgery]. Neurochirurgie 2004;50(2–3 Pt 2):383–93.

[21] Friedman RA, Brackmann DE, Hitselberger WE, et al. Surgical salvage after failed irradiation for vestibular schwannoma. Laryngoscope 2005;115(10):1827–32.

[22] Noren G, Arndt J, Hindmarsh T. Stereotactic radiosurgery in cases of acoustic neurinoma: further experiences. Neurosurgery 1983;13(1):12–22.

[23] Kondziolka D, Lunsford LD, Flickinger JC. Comparison of management options for patients with acoustic neuromas. Neurosurg Focus 2003;14(5):e1.

[24] Lunsford LD, Niranjan A, Flickinger JC, et al. Radiosurgery of vestibular schwannomas: summary of experience in 829 cases. J Neurosurg 2005;102(Suppl):195–9.

[25] McEvoy AW, Kitchen ND. Rapid enlargement of a vestibular schwannoma following gamma knife treatment. Minim Invasive Neurosurg 2003;46(4):254–6.

[26] Sanna M, Falcioni M, Taibah A, et al. Treatment of residual vestibular schwannoma. Otol Neurotol 2002;23(6):980–7.

[27] Mueller DP, Gantz BJ, Dolan KD. Gadolinium-enhanced MR of the postoperative internal auditory canal following acoustic neuroma resection via the middle fossa approach. AJNR Am J Neuroradiol 1992;13(1):197–200.

[28] Elster AD, DiPersio DA. Cranial postoperative site: assessment with contrast-enhanced MR imaging. Radiology 1990;174(1):93–8.

[29] Roberson JB Jr, Brackmann DE, Hitselberger WE. Acoustic neuroma recurrence after suboccipital resection: management with translabyrinthine resection. Am J Otol 1996;17(2):307–11.

[30] Ciric I, Zhao JC, Rosenblatt S, et al. Suboccipital retrosigmoid approach for removal of vestibular schwannomas: facial nerve function and hearing preservation. Neurosurgery 2005;56(3):560–70 [discussion: 70].

ELSEVIER
SAUNDERS

Otolaryngol Clin N Am
39 (2006) 763–782

OTOLARYNGOLOGIC
CLINICS
OF NORTH AMERICA

Revision Glomus Tumor Surgery

Mario Sanna, MD[a],*, Giuseppe De Donato, MD[a],
Paolo Piazza, MD[b], Maurizio Falcioni, MD[a]

[a]*Gruppo Otologico, via Emmanueli 42, 29100, Piacenza, Italy*
[b]*Department of Neuroradiology, University of Parma, via Abbeveratoia, 43100, Parma, Italy*

Surgical removal of tympano-jugular paragangliomas (TJP) has always been a difficult task for the skull base surgeon. The standardization of the infratemporal fossa type A approach by Ugo Fisch [1] in 1978 was a milestone in the treatment of these lesions, as well as the development of preoperative interventional radiologic techniques like preoperative embolization [2] and internal carotid artery (ICA) preoperative treatment [2–4]. These terrific improvements made possible the resection of tumors considered inoperable until a few years ago. However, removal of this kind of lesion remains a demanding task. Alternative treatments proposed in the literature include a "wait and see" policy [5], conventional radiotherapy [6,7], and, more recently, stereotactic radiotherapy, alone or in association with removal of the middle ear component of the tumor [8–11].

"Wait and see" is based on the general belief that TJPs are benign, slow-growing lesions. Unfortunately, the course of at least one subgroup of these large tumors, usually affecting younger patients, seems completely different [12,13]. Therefore, this policy is recommended currently only in select cases, mainly those of elderly patients with intact lower cranial nerve function.

Conventional radiotherapy has no direct effect on the tumoral cells, producing only fibrosis of the vessels supplying the tumor [6,7,14]. Recurrences are also documented [13]. In addition, potentially life-threatening complications like osteoradionecrosis and induction of malignancy have been reported [15,16].

No large series treated with stereotactic radiotherapy exists to confirm its effectiveness in long-term follow-up. The majority of recurrences seem to occur at least 5 years after surgical removal. Stereotactic radiotherapy is suggested mainly for small TJPs confined to the jugular bulb [11]. However, it

* Corresponding author.
E-mail address: mario.sanna@gruppootologico.it (M. Sanna).

0030-6665/06/$ - see front matter © 2006 Elsevier Inc. All rights reserved.
doi:10.1016/j.otc.2006.04.004
oto.theclinics.com

does not seem indicated in large lesions with extensive bone infiltration, where its effects are questionable and the risks of osteoradionecrosis may be comparable to those of conventional radiotherapy.

For these reasons, microsurgery remains the preferred treatment modality in most cases, at least in patients with a life expectancy of more than 20 years, even with the risk of recurrence.

The aim of this article is to analyze the reasons for these recurrences, in an attempt to determine the steps that can be adopted to reduce their number. In addition, surgical problems encountered when operating on recurrent TJPs are evaluated together with the solutions currently adopted at the Gruppo Otologico [17,18]. This evaluation is based on the experience acquired through the surgical removal of 81 TJPs from 1985 to November 2005 (the number does not include those cases of the senior author, MS, operated on in another institution).

Reasons for recurrence and steps to reduce their number

Incomplete removal may result from unpredicted intraoperative problems that made it impossible to complete the surgery, or from a planned partial or subtotal operation. However, during follow-up, recurrences sometimes appear, even in cases originally classified as successful gross total removal. Most of these cases are the result of incorrect preoperative evaluation and planning, and may be managed during a second stage after proper preoperative assessment.

Planned partial removal has been recommended strongly, especially in recent years [19], supported by the general belief that TJPs are benign slow-growing lesions. This solution has gained consensus among the skull base community. Indications for a planned partial removal should be evaluated accurately; the temporary benefit to the patient of avoiding a facial nerve (FN) weakness, hearing loss, or a lower cranial nerve palsy should be balanced against the possibility that, because of the infiltrating nature of TJPs, tumoral remnants may spread along the dural surfaces (Fig. 1) and the spongy bone, reaching areas where they become unresectable. In fact, large lesions affecting young patients usually show a particularly aggressive pattern, with a high recurrence rate. The authors have seen two patients operated on in other institutions who died because of recurrent disease: the first one refused an additional revision surgery after multiple attempts to control the tumor through conservative operations; the second died of intracranial complications 2 days before the planned preoperative embolization and surgery.

The authors currently plan a partial removal only in rare cases, such as those with cavernous sinus involvement. Small remnants, especially when located intradurally, may be treated by stereotactic radiotherapy, even if, currently, no long-term follow-up data regarding the fate of these patients are available.

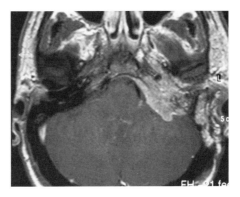

Fig. 1. MRI; recurrent TJP. Involvement of the dura by tumoral infiltration is visible along the posterior surface of the temporal bone, reaching the petro-clival junction.

Another selective indication for partial removal is in elderly patients managed initially by a "wait and see" policy who start to complain of recurrent otorrhagia; in these cases the removal should be limited to the middle ear and mastoid components.

The most common reasons for a tumor recurrence after a presumed gross total removal in the presence of a TJP are

- Surgeon's inexperience
- Incorrect preoperative evaluation and planning
- Extensive bone infiltration
- Incomplete carotid artery management
- No execution of FN rerouting
- Attempted preservation of the lower cranial nerves when involved
- Undetected dural infiltration
- Excessive bleeding during surgery

Surgeon's inexperience

This demanding surgery should take place only in selected referral centers because a surgeon's inexperience may result in not only a higher recurrence rate, but also an increased postoperative morbidity.

Incorrect preoperative evaluation and planning

Routine preoperative work-up must always include an accurate radiologic evaluation that is best accomplished through high resolution CT, high field MRI, magnetic resonance angiography (MRA) and intra-arterial transfemoral digital subtraction angiography.

All these radiologic examinations together help in reaching the correct diagnosis and in classifying the tumor according to the more frequently used classifications. The authors adopted the Fisch classification [20] since 1988.

However, an integration with the Moret classification [21], which categorizes the TJPs from an angiographic point of view, has improved radiologic evaluation for surgical planning.

The most common areas of incorrect preoperative evaluation include differentiation between class B and C tumors, and evaluation of the ICA and intradural spaces involvement. The problems related to the ICA and the dural involvement are discussed later.

Careful evaluation of the bony separation between the hypotympanum and the jugular bulb usually enables the surgeon to differentiate between class B and class C paragangliomas and select the appropriate approach. However, the authors have two cases in their series in which, because of an incorrect preoperative evaluation, the patient underwent a middle ear surgery to remove a class B paraganglioma and during surgery an invasion of the jugular bulb was discovered. A residual tumor was therefore left at the level of the jugular bulb, giving rise to a recurrence.

Incorrect planning may also occur when considering the possible involvement of anatomic areas usually spared, such as the inner ear, the occipital condyle, and, rarely, the vertebral artery. All these structures need careful preoperative assessment to determine whether they need to be sacrificed to reach the goal of total removal. Once, in the authors' series, a rare extension of TJP along the extracranial course of the left vertebral artery required the preoperative occlusion of the artery itself; it was finally removed during a second stage, through an extreme lateral approach. Similar cases have been reported in the literature [13].

Extensive bone infiltration

Aggressive bone infiltration, as confirmed by the characteristic pattern of bony erosion detectable on CT (Fig. 2), is a particular feature of TJP, even if different statements are present in the literature [9]. Infiltration is particularly frequent at the level of the spongy bone of the petrous apex. Sometimes, it is difficult to distinguish between normal and infiltrated bone, both in the preoperative scans and during surgery. For this reason, it is strongly advisable to drill out as much bone as possible at the level of the petrous apex, medial to the vertical and, if necessary, the horizontal portion of the ICA [22]. When required, the ICA may also be mobilized partially (Fig. 3). A residual lesion at this level may engulf the artery, making revision surgery extremely difficult. The same is true for the tympanic bone, often infiltrated in a medial to lateral direction, sometimes causing the classic "rising sun" otoscopic appearance [23]. Any attempt to preserve the external auditory canal may result in incomplete removal.

Incomplete carotid artery management

ICA involvement in TJPs occurs frequently, and in the authors' series some kind of artery treatment was required in 91% of cases, ranging from

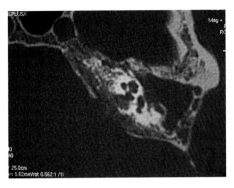

Fig. 2. CT, same patient as Fig. 1. The characteristic irregular patter of bony erosion is evident along the medial surface of the temporal bone, making it difficult to distinguish between infiltrated and noninfiltrated bone at the level of the petrous apex.

simple skeletonization to subadventitial dissection or removal after preoperative occlusion (Fig. 4). In 5 out of 7 cases, histopathologic examination of the removed adventitia indicated tumor infiltration. Some of the most experienced surgeons have reported intraoperative injury to the ICA, with subsequent complications like massive stroke and death [12,24]. Therefore, carotid involvement must be evaluated carefully during the preoperative work-up to select the correct treatment.

Indications for interventional radiologic preoperative treatment of the ICA include engulfment by the tumor by more than 270° as shown by MRI and MRA, evidence of stenosis of the arterial lumen or arterial wall irregularities on the arteriography, class C3 and C4 TJPs whereby the tumor should be dissected from the genu or the horizontal portion, and extensive blood supply from branches of the ICA. Treatment is mandatory in recurrent or postradiation cases.

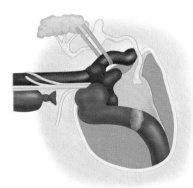

Fig. 3. To completely remove the infiltrated bone of the carotid canal, partial dislocation of the ICA may be required.

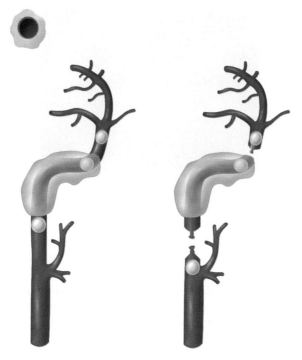

Fig. 4. Permanent occlusion of the ICA is achieved by means of positioning one balloon at the level of the cervical portion and two at the level of the anterior foramen lacerum and precavernous segment. Intraoperatively, after additional ligation at the level of the cervical portion, the intrapetrous carotid artery can be removed completely with the tumor.

If preoperative angiography shows adequate collateral circulation through the circle of Willis, a balloon test occlusion of the ICA with clinical and angiographic tolerance, followed by permanent balloon occlusion [25], is considered the simplest and most effective procedure. However, this procedure is not risk free, and, although rare, complications can be serious [3]. In addition, it cannot be used in cases of inadequate collateral circulation.

The bypass of the ICA [26] has been considered the only option in cases of inadequate collateral circulation, but, regardless of the technique used, this procedure is a major surgical operation and carries a relatively high risk of stenosis, thrombo-embolism, and occlusion [27,28]. Two out of three cases in the authors' paraganglioma series treated by means of ICA by-pass resulted in failure, with occlusion of the by-pass.

The recent introduction of preoperative stenting has made more aggressive carotid dissection feasible (Fig. 5), decreasing significantly the related possible risks, and greatly reducing the need for permanent balloon occlusion. In addition, when the tumor infiltrates the wall of the artery, it may derive abundant blood supply directly from the ICA; in such situations

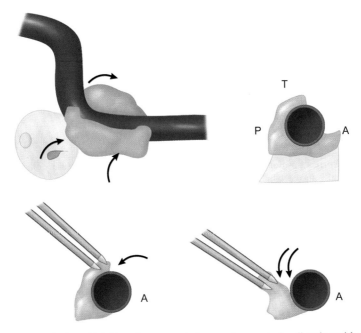

Fig. 5. Careful subadventitial dissection proceeds in an antero-posterior direction with the help of bipolar cautery and microscissors. A, anterior; P, posterior; T, tumor.

positioning of the stent also contributes to preoperative devascularization of the lesion.

Currently, the authors consider the Xpert stent (Abbot Vascular Laboratories, Dublin, Ireland) the most suitable for stenting both the cervical and intratemporal portions of the ICA because of its diameter, length, and flexibility. This stent is available in various diameters (4 or 5 mm) and lengths (20, 30, or 40 mm) that are selected carefully, tailoring the procedure to each patient. In some cases, however, inserting the Xpert stent in the petrous portion of the ICA has been impossible, so the authors were forced to choose a softer and more fragile Neuroform 3 stent (Boston Scientific, Fremont, California), with a diameter of 4 mm and length of 30 mm.

The risk of stent thrombosis is still present and pre- and poststenting antiplatelet therapy should be continued for life. In the authors' practice, patients to be stented are started on 250 mg oral ticlopidine twice a day and 100 mg salicylate daily, 1 week before the insertion of the stent. This combination is continued for 1 month after the insertion of the stent. From this point onwards, oral salicylate is continued for life. The only interruption of this regimen is during the perioperative period (from 1 week before to 1 week after surgery), when it is replaced by low molecular weight heparin.

To reduce the risk of injuring the ICA at its junction with the tumor, the authors believe that at least a 5 to 10 mm of tumor-free ICA should be

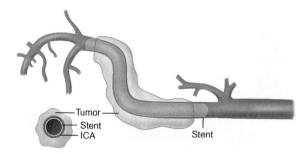

Fig. 6. The correct position of the stent should reach at least 5 to 10 mm of tumor-free ICA, both proximally and distally.

reinforced with the stent, both proximally and distally (Fig. 6). To achieve this, it might be necessary to insert two or even three stents. A stent is placed 4 to 6 weeks before the planned date of the operation to allow a stabilized neointimal lining to form on the luminal surface of the stent, as shown in the histopathologic examination at autopsy by Toma and colleagues [29].

The assessment of the long-term patency of the stented ICA is performed by Doppler ultrasonography. In the authors' series, there have been no cases showing signs of stenosis or occlusion of the stented segment of the ICA.

Permanent occlusion should be considered when it is impossible to insert the stent in the desired position because of coiling and kinking of the cervical portion of the ICA, or when there is extensive blood supply from the petrous and cavernous branches of the ICA to the tumor.

No execution of facial nerve rerouting

A less aggressive treatment, the so-called "fallopian bridge technique [30]," has been advocated recently by some investigators because it makes possible the removal of C1 and C2 TJPs without any need to dislocate the FN and remove the external and middle ear. In the authors' opinion, when treating vascular lesions, this "conservative" approach does not allow any control of the area of the lesion's origin or of the ICA (Fig. 7). As a consequence, this treatment will probably produce more recurrences in following years. Always, the goal of preserving as many functions as possible should be considered during the preoperative planning; however, skull base surgeons must also be aware of the extreme aggressiveness of this kind of lesion. An initial "conservative" surgery may produce a spread of the lesion to areas where it becomes very difficult to manage. Temporary FN palsy, with a high percentage of recovery to grade I or II at 1 year (65.8% in the authors' series, ranging from 51% and 95% in the literature) [17,31–33], and conductive hearing loss are the price to be paid for attempting total removal, which the authors consider the correct goal, at least in young patients. In their series, the authors have two patients who were operated on in other centers

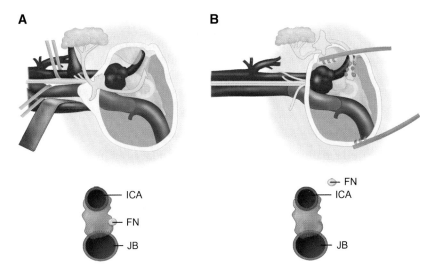

Fig. 7. (*A*) The FN left in place impedes adequate control of the carotid artery and the surrounding tumor. (*B*) Once the FN has been rerouted, direct control of the area of the ICA is possible.

without FN rerouting and who presented a recurrence a few years later (Fig. 8). Another patient is currently completing the preoperative work-up.

Attempted preservation of the lower cranial nerves when involved

For the same reason, it is not advisable to attempt to preserve the anatomic integrity of the lower cranial nerves when there is tumor involvement, which usually occurs when the lesion infiltrates the medial wall of the jugular bulb. In the authors' experience, dissection of the involved nerves has always resulted in a complete palsy, with the additional risk of leaving some tumoral remnants medial to the jugular foramen.

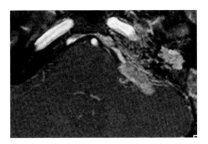

Fig. 8. MRI, same patient as Figs. 1 and 2. After three attempts at removal through a "conservative" approach without FN rerouting, a tumor recurrence is still present, with complete engulfment of the horizontal portion of the ICA.

Undetected dural infiltration

It is not always possible to detect a dural involvement clearly from the preoperative scans. Even if a large intradural component is not usual in this kind of lesion, dural infiltration is particularly common. Possible dural infiltrations managed conservatively may result in intradural recurrences after some years.

Excessive bleeding during surgery

Because of the nature of vascular lesions, standardized treatment of TJPs currently includes preoperative embolization to reduce intraoperative bleeding. The bleeding may represent not only an additional risk for the patient, but also a reason for incomplete tumor resection, because of the impossibility of perfectly controlling the surgical field. Embolization is extremely important and complete control of the intraoperative bleeding needs correct surgical strategy.

Delayed ligation of the jugular vein into the neck and extensive bone drilling before starting tumor resection may also reduce excessive bleeding. In fact, ligation of the jugular vein during the first steps of the surgery may produce a venous stasis (if the vein is still patent) with increased bleeding in the surgical field. The vein should be isolated early but its ligation delayed until after the occlusion of the sigmoid sinus.

Other possible origins of bleeding are the orifices of the inferior petrosal sinus and the condylar vein, often not occluded by the tumor extensions. Packing of the vessels is usually required to stop the bleeding, taking into account that the more common location of the orifice of the inferior petrosal sinus is at the level of the medial wall of the jugular bulb, in close relationship with the lower cranial nerves. Connection of the inferior petrosal sinus directly with the jugular vein is encountered less frequently.

Intratumoral bleeding is very difficult to control. It is advisable to completely dissect the lesion from its bony bounders and only then, after cauterization of the tumoral surface, start the TJP removal. Excessive bleeding makes the already difficult identification of the limits of the lesion much more problematic, particularly at the level of the petrous apex bone.

A detailed list of recurrences treated at the authors' center is reported in Tables 1 and 2.

Illustrative case 1 (V.P.)

In October 1996, a 32-year-old woman came to the authors' attention because she was affected by a TJP. In addition to the usual symptoms, the patient complained of a VI cranial nerve palsy, produced by tumor invasion of the Dorello's canal. The diagnostic work-up classified the lesion as a C4 Di2. The ICA appeared largely involved (Fig. 9); however, the preoperative occlusion test failed because of the absence of contralateral compensation. A staged subtotal removal was planned, leaving some tumor remnants at

Table 1
Recurrences in patients operated at Gruppo Otologico

Patient	Class	1st operation	Recurrence (location)	Revision	Follow-up
Z.R.	C2	1990 IFT-A, no rerouting	1996 petrous apex, jugular foramen, medial to ICA	Refused	2003 growth; refused surgery
A.L.	C3 Di1	1996 IFT-A + TLA (I stage) ICA: balloon occlusion & removal 1997 MTCA + sural graft (II stage)	1997 foramen magnum, occipital condyle, clivus	Repeated percutaneous embolizations with Hystoacryl	2004 growth
P.G.	C2 Di2	1994 IFT-A (I stage) 1995 extreme lateral (II stage)	1998 prevertebral spaces, foramen magnum - C2	2004 IFT (partial removal) ICA: stent	2005 evaluation for further revision
V.P.[a]	C4 Di2	1997 IFT-A (I stage) 1998 TLA + petrooccipital (II stage) gamma knife (cavernous sinus)	2001 ICA	2004 IFT-A (I stage) ICA: stent 2005 petrooccipital (II stage)	2005 cavernous sinus (no growth)

Abbreviations: IFT-A, infratemporal type A; MTCA, modified transcochlear approach; TLA, translabyrinthine approach.

[a] Illustrative case 1.

the level of the ICA to avoid the risk of intraoperative artery rupture, and at the level of the cavernous sinus to maintain the occular motility. After preoperative embolization, the first stage was performed through an infratemporal type A approach. As planned, the intradural component and some tumor around the ICA were left in place.

After a few months, the patient underwent a new embolization and the planned second stage. At that time, the postoperative FN palsy had recovered to grade II. During surgery, the approach was extended with a labyrinthectomy and removal of the cochlea. Further bone removal was achieved medial to the ICA and at the level of the lateral portion of the occipital condyle. All the dura covering the posterior surface of the petrous bone appeared infiltrated by the tumor and was removed as far as the entrance of the Dorello's canal. The VI cranial nerve, already paralyzed, was sacrificed because it was engulfed completely by the lesion. The disease was also removed from the Meckel's cave while avoiding entering the cavernous sinus,

Table 2
Recurrences operated in other centers and revisioned at Gruppo Otologico

Patient	Class	1st operation	Recurrence (location)	Revision	Follow-up
A.E.[a]	C4 Di1	1992 cervical approach (vagal paraganglioma?) intraoperative rupture of the ICA (suture)	1998 jugular foramen, ICA, petrous apex, occipital condyle, cavernous sinus	1999 IFT-A ICA: by-pass; balloon occlusion + removal gamma knife	2006 no evidence of recurrence
B.C.	C2 De2	1986 IFT-A; no rerouting	1994 ICA	1994 IFT-A	2005 free of disease
C.F.	C3 Di1	1990 occipital transigmoid 1993 revision	1999 jugular foramen, ICA, occipital condyle	2002 IFT-A (I stage) ICA: ballon occlusion + removal 2003 petrooccipital approach (II stage)	2003 residual tumor in the clivus (1 cm)
O.I.	Ce Di1	1983 radical mastoidectomy	1996 IAC, petrous apex, occipital condyle, ICA	1996 IFT-A + TLA ICA: balloon occlusion + removal	2005 free of disease
V.A.	C2	2004 radical cavity	2005 jugular foramen, ICA, petrous apex, occipital condyle	2005 IFT-A ICA: dissection	contralateral carotid body paraganglioma recently operated

Abbreviations: IFT-A, infratemporal type A; TLA, translabyrinthine approach.
a Illustrative case 2.

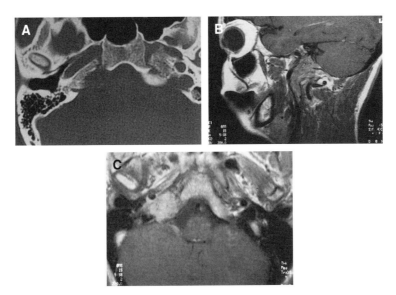

Fig. 9. (*A*) CT scan showing bone erosion medial to the horizontal segment of the intrapetrous ICA. (*B*) Sagittal MRI showing the extension of the tumor into the neck and the involvement of the ICA. (*C*) Involvement of the ICA is best appreciated on axial images.

as preoperatively planned. In the postoperative period, the FN function deteriorated to grade IV. A complementary treatment by means of stereotactic radiotherapy was performed for the cavernous sinus involvement. Radiologic controls on January 1999 showed no tumor growth of the residual lesion in the cavernous sinus, whereas residual lesion was detectable at the level of the ICA. However, in the following controls, a recurrent lesion became more and more evident around the ICA (Fig. 10); it was managed conservatively because of the impossibility of closing the artery as well. In 2003, new opportunities arose, thanks to the possibility of using a stent to reinforce the arterial walls of the ICA. After the stent was positioned (Fig. 11), the patient underwent a new embolization and surgery through

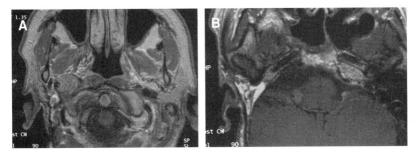

Fig. 10. (*A*) Postoperative MRI showing a recurrent lesion engulfing the carotid artery at the entrance to the skull base. (*B*) The recurrent lesion is still visible at the level of the carotid genu.

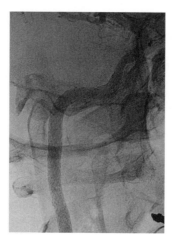

Fig. 11. Radiologic confirmation of the correct position of the stent is achieved easily through conventional radiographs.

the same approach. The artery was engulfed at 360° and its treatment required an extensive subadventitial dissection along all the vertical and horizontal segments. The carotid canal was drilled off to the anterior foramen lacerum (Fig. 12). To avoid postoperative cerebrospinal leak, the recurrent intradural lesion was left in place.

In June 2005, the final removal of this last component was planned, with resection of the remaining portion of the occipital condyle, the location of an additional recurrence. So far, no growth of the cavernous sinus remnant has been detected. FN function is currently grade II.

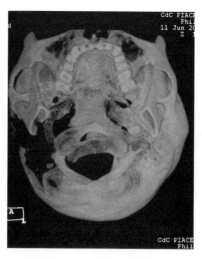

Fig. 12. 3D reconstruction on CT shows the extent of bone removal reaching the area of the foramen lacerum.

Illustrative case 2 (A.E.)

In 1992, a 24-year-old man was operated on at another center using a lat-ero-cervical approach for a right-sided lesion diagnosed as a vagal paragan-glioma. During dissection of the ICA, a tear of the artery wall was managed by suture.

In 1998, after the appearance of a pulsatile tinnitus and a sudden hearing loss, radiologic investigation detected a recurrence at the level of the jugular foramen (Fig. 13). The new data made it probable that the diagnosis of va-gal paraganglioma had not been correct, or was at least incomplete; the tu-mor had probably been a TJP from the beginning, alone or associated with a vagal paraganglioma. Because of the engulfment of the ICA, and taking into consideration the rupture that occurred during the first surgery, an at-tempt to dissect the artery was considered too risky. Because of the patient's young age, prophylactic external-internal carotid artery by-pass was per-formed in another center. The patient was then seen at the authors' center where a new angiography showed occlusion of the by-pass. Following good tolerance at the occlusion test, the patient underwent a permanent bal-loon occlusion of the ICA without complications.

In July 1999, he was operated on again to remove the recurrent lesion through an infratemporal type A approach with resection of the ICA from the neck to the anterior foramen lacerum. Tumor infiltration was found in the petrous apex to the clivus and the occipital condyle. A small remnant was left at the level of the cavernous sinus.

The postoperative period was uneventful. The suspect remnant was treated with gamma knife. As of the last follow-up (2006) the postoperative scans did not show any further recurrence (Fig. 14).

Surgical problems in recurrent tympano-jugular paragangliomas

The first problem related to unexpected TJP recurrence is its early radio-logic detection. Postoperative scans of the skull base (both MRI and CT) are

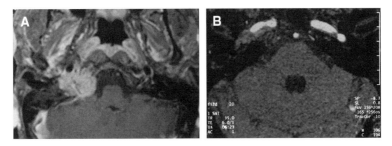

Fig. 13. (*A*) On axial MRI it is possible to detect the relationship between tumor and carotid artery, with the latter engulfed for more than 270°. (*B*) Carotid artery engulfment is also present at the level of the horizontal portion.

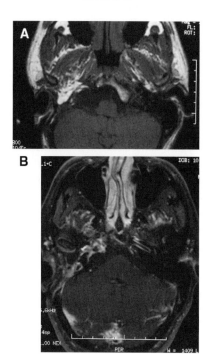

Fig. 14. (*A*) Postoperative MRI allows confirmation of total tumor removal. Note the absence of the carotid artery, surgically removed after preoperative occlusion. (*B*) Total tumor removal and absence of the carotid artery may also be appreciated on higher cuts.

often difficult to interpret and recurrences are not identified clearly until they have already reached considerable size. On the contrary, digital angiography, even if able to detect smaller lesions, is an invasive technique and not advisable for routine follow-up. However, to reduce the rate of delayed detection of tumoral recurrence, the possibility of performing a control angiography 5 years after surgery (in addition to the routine follow-up examination with MRI and CT) may be discussed with the patient. In every case, the difficulty of detecting the anatomic limit of the recurrence should indicate to the surgeon that he may be dealing with a lesion larger than on the scan.

When a surgical removal is planned, the surgeon should be aware of the additional difficulties associated with significant reduction of available landmarks, especially when, during the first surgery, a labyrinthectomy was added to the main approach. From experience acquired staging intradural lesions, the authors prefer to leave at least some portions of the labyrinth in order to have some reliable bony landmarks in case of recurrent lesion. Because of this, the authors do not agree with Brackmann [34], who advises repositioning of the FN at the end of the surgery. This repositioning leaves the nerve in the middle of the residual cavity, engulfed by the scar tissue resulting from fat obliteration, making its identification difficult in any revision surgery. On the contrary, the FN has to be left anteriorly dislodged, in an area in which the recurrence never occurs.

In patients who have already experienced radiotherapy or an aggressive surgery with some kind of ICA treatment, the carotid wall is usually more fragile. Precautional interventional neuroradiologic measures should be taken to reduce the risk of a perioperative tear.

Surgical solutions in recurrent tympano-jugular paragangliomas

No definitive solutions exist for the difficult problems related to revision surgery for recurrent TJPs. The authors prefer the very aggressive approach of adopting the infratemporal type A in every case, with or without trans-labyrinthine extension. The critical points seem to be the FN, ICA and the lower cranial nerves.

The FN must be rerouted in all cases if it has been left in place during the first surgery, to control the critical area corresponding to the entrance of the ICA and the jugular vein into the skull base. Naturally, in the presence of a recurrent lesion, a skeletonized FN remains protected only by a tiny shell of bone and is at higher risk of infiltration, and the same is true in the presence of partial (short) anterior rerouting [32]. In addition, when the FN has remained suspended on a thin fallopian bridge, its dislocation is far more difficult because of the constant risk of fracture of the bony support, with consequent interruption of the FN. In the case of tumoral infiltration confined to the epineurium, it is advisable to reroute the nerve first, and, only at the end of the procedure, when the nerve is already in place, to peel the epineurium carefully. Reversing the two steps endangers the integrity of the FN because a nerve denudated of its epineurium is much more fragile during the maneuvers required to reroute it.

In most of the surgical cases at the Gruppo Otologico, the recurrence developed around the ICA (see Table 1), suggesting that our initial surgery, even if aggressive, was not enough. When dealing with a recurrent lesion at the level of the ICA, interventional neuroradiologic preoperative treatment is almost always mandatory. The availability of stent insertion has limited the necessity of permanent balloon occlusion of the ICA to selected cases. The presence of a stent offers the surgeon the possibility of a more aggressive subadventitial dissection, especially in cases already treated, where the artery wall may be more fragile. So far, the authors have encountered only one case in which it was impossible to introduce the stent, because of a kinking of the artery at the entrance into the skull. Functional angiographic evaluation showed inadequate collateral circulation through the circle of Willis, so that, because of the extensive carotid involvement, the patient underwent a carotid by-pass, followed by permanent balloon occlusion of the ICA.

When the surgical field has been radiated previously or the artery already has been dissected partially during the first surgery, or in cases with extensive blood supply from the ICA branches, carotid removal after permanent occlusion, when feasible, still seems the safest option.

All the bone surrounding the recurrence should be drilled out aggressively, keeping in mind that the infiltration is often more extensive than that visible on the scans. Drilling is only stopped when the surgeon is reasonably sure he has removed all the potentially infiltrated bone and can visualize normal bone.

The surgeon should strike a balance between lower cranial nerve preservation and radical removal. Usually, infiltration of the medial wall of the jugular bulb makes it very difficult, if not impossible, to save the nerve function and increases the risk of a recurrence. The authors do not hesitate to sacrifice the nerves when there is a recurrence with infiltration of the medial wall of the jugular bulb. Sacrifice of the still functioning nerves may require a prolonged rehabilitation, often accompanied by surgical correction like thyroplasty or vocal cord augmentation, but it is usually well tolerated by young patients.

Summary

Despite their aggressive stance, so far the authors have experienced five recurrences out of 81 TJPs surgically treated, which corresponds to 6.2%. This percentage is probably higher in centers that take a much more conservative approach.

They strongly advocate using the infratemporal fossa approach type A in every case of TJP, because FN rerouting is key in reaching the area of the ICA, where recurrence is most likely to occur. When corrected, accomplished anterior FN rerouting allows a recovery to a grade I or II function at 1 year in around 70% of the cases. Preservation of the lower cranial nerve function is not feasible in the presence of tumor infiltration of the medial wall of the jugular bulb; any attempt at nerve dissection increases the risk of leaving some tumor remnants.

Correct management of the ICA, including preoperative stent insertion or preoperative permanent balloon occlusion, represents, in the authors' opinion, the fundamental step when dealing with recurrent TJPs. Because of the tumor tendency to infiltrate the bony structures, aggressive drilling of the temporal bone is also advised.

Although preservation of neurologic functions has been stressed correctly during recent years, this must be balanced against the fact that patients affected by resultant uncontrolled recurrences still die because of this disease.

References

[1] Fisch U. The infratemporal fossa approach to tumors of the temporal bone and base of the skull. J Laryngol Otol 1978;92:949–67.

[2] Valavanis A. Preoperative embolization of the head and neck: indications, patient selection, goals, and precautions. AJNR Am J Neuroradiol 1986;7(5):943–52.

[3] Sanna M, Piazza P, Di Trapani G, et al. Management of the internal carotid artery in tumors of the lateral skull base: preoperative permanent balloon occlusion without reconstruction. Otol Neurotol 2004;25(6):998–1005.

[4] Sanna M, Khrais T, Piazza P, et al. Stent of the internal carotid artery for the management of jugular paragangliomas. Laryngoscope, in press.

[5] van der Mey AG, Frijns JH, Cornelisse CJ, et al. Does intervention improve the natural course of glomus tumors? A series of 108 patients seen in a 32-year period. Ann Otol Rhinol Laryngol 1992;101(8):635–42.

[6] Carrasco V, Rosenman J. Radiation therapy of glomus jugulare tumors. Laryngoscope 1993;103(Suppl 60):23–7.

[7] Hawthorne MR, Makek MS, Harris JP, et al. The histopatological and clinical features of irradiated and nonirradiated temporal paragangliomas. Laryngoscope 1988;98:325–31.

[8] Pollock BE. Stereotactic radiosurgery in patients with glomus jugulare tumors. Neurosurg Focus 2004;17:63–7.

[9] Lim M, Gibbs IC, Adler JR, et al. Efficacy and safety of stereotactic radiosurgery for glomus jugulare tumors. Neurosurg Focus 2004;17:68–72.

[10] Jordan JA, Roland PS, McManus C, et al. Stereotactic radiosurgery for glomus jugulare tumors. Laryngoscope 2000;110:35–8.

[11] Willen SN, Einstein DB, Maciunas RJ, et al. Treatment of glomus jugulare tumors in patients with advanced age: planned limited surgical resection followed by staged gamma knife radiosurgery: a preliminary report. Otol Neurotol 2005;26:1229–34.

[12] Al-mefty O, Teixeira A. Complex tumors of the glomus jugulare: criteria, treatment, and outcome. J Neurosurg 2002;97:1356–66.

[13] Patel SJ, Sekhar LN, Cass SP, et al. Combined approach for resection of extensive glomus jugulare tumors. J Neurosurg 1994;80:1026–38.

[14] Brackmann DE, House WF, Terry R, et al. Glomus jugulare tumors: effect of irradiation. Trans Am Acad Ophthalmol Otolaryngol 1972;76(6):1423–31.

[15] Cole JM, Beiler D. Long-term results of treatment for glomus jugulare and glomus vagale tumors. Laryngoscope 1994;104:1461–5.

[16] Lalwani AK, Jackler RK, Gutin PH. Lethal fibrosarcoma complicating radiation therapy for benign glomus jugulare tumor. Am J Otol 1993;14:398–402.

[17] Sanna M, Jain Y, De Donato G, et al. Management of jugular paragangliomas: the Gruppo Otologico experience. Otol Neurotol 2004;25(5):797–804.

[18] Sanna M, De Donato G, Russo A, et al. Middle ear and skull base glomus tumors: tympanic and tympanojugular paragangliomas. In: Wiet RJ, editor. Ear and temporal bone surgery: minimizing risks and complications. New York: Thieme; 222–234 (in press).

[19] Oghalai JS, Leung MK, Jackler RK, et al. Transjugular craniotomy for the management of jugular foramen tumors with intracranial extension. Otol Neurotol 2004;25:570–9.

[20] Fisch U, Mattox D. Microsurgery of the skull base. New York: Thieme; 1988.

[21] Moret J, Lasjaunias P, Theron J. Vascular compartments and territories of timpano-jugular glomic tumors. J Belge Radiol 1980;63:321–37.

[22] Sanna M, Saleh E, Russo A, et al. Atlas of temporal bone and skull base surgery. Stuttgart/New York: Georg Thieme Verlag; 1995. p. 132–145.

[23] Sanna M, Russo A, De Donato G, et al. Color atlas of otoscopy (2nd edition). Stuttgart/New York: Georg Thieme Verlag; 2002.

[24] Jackson G, Kaylie D, Coppit G, et al. Glomus jugulare tumors with intracranial extension. Neurosurg Focus. 2004;17:45–50.

[25] Zane RS, Aeschbacher P, Moll C, et al. Carotid occlusion without reconstruction: a safe surgical option in selected patients. Am J Otol 1995;16:353–9.

[26] Urken ML, Biller HF, Haimov M. Intratemporal carotid artery bypass in resection of a base of skull tumor. Laryngoscope 1985;95(12):1472–7.

[27] Chazono H, Okamoto Y, Matsuzaki Z, et al. Extracranial-intracranial bypass for recon-
     struction of internal carotid artery in the management of head and neck cancer. Ann Vasc
     Surg 2003;17(3):260–5.
[28] Roddy SP, Darling RC 3rd, et al. Choice of material for internal carotid artery bypass graft-
     ing: vein or prosthetic? Analysis of 44 procedures. Cardiovasc Surg 2002;10(6):540–4.
[29] Toma N, Matsushima S, Murao K, et al. Histopathological findings in a human carotid ar-
     tery after stent implantation. Case report. J Neurosurg 2003;98(1):199–204.
[30] Pensak ML, Jackler RK. Removal of jugular foramen tumors: the fallopian bridge tech-
     nique. Otolaryngol Head Neck Surg 1997;117:586–91.
[31] Russo A, Piccirillo E, De Donato G, et al. Anterior and posterior facial nerve rerouting:
     a comparative study. Skull Base 2003;13(3):123–30.
[32] Parhizkar N, Hiltzik DH, Selesnick SH. Facial nerve rerouting in skull base surgery. Otolar-
     yngol Clin N am 2005;38:685–710.
[33] Selesnick SH, Abraham MT, Carew JF. Rerouting of the intratemporal facial nerve: an anal-
     ysis of the literature. Am J Otol 1996;17:793–805.
[34] Brackmann DE. The facial nerve in infratemporal approach. Otolaryngol Head Neck Surg
     1987;97:15–7.

ELSEVIER
SAUNDERS

Otolaryngol Clin N Am
39 (2006) 783–799

OTOLARYNGOLOGIC
CLINICS
OF NORTH AMERICA

The Challenges of Revision Skull Base Surgery

Anh Nguyen-Huynh, MD, PhD*,
Nikolas H. Blevins, MD, Robert K. Jackler, MD

*Department of Otolaryngology–Head & Neck Surgery,
Stanford University School of Medicine, 801 Welch Road, Stanford, CA 94305-5739, USA*

The complex anatomy of the posterolateral skull base and its high density of vital neurovascular structures often preclude complete resection of tumors involving this region. Surgeons often leave remnants of tumor behind, either knowingly, to avoid iatrogenic injury, or as a consequence of suboptimal exposure. As a result, neurotologic surgeons are often faced with persistent or recurrent disease that requires careful evaluation for revision surgery.

The increasing use of radiotherapy also affects the surgical management of skull base tumors. On the one hand, the efficacy of postoperative adjuvant radiotherapy makes it possible to perform intentional subtotal resection to preserve function while controlling tumor growth. On the other hand, the rise of radiotherapy as a primary treatment will give rise to more patients with radiation failures, whose salvage surgeries will have their own set of challenges.

This article discusses general considerations in the diagnosis and management of recurrent skull base tumors, and specific issues pertaining to meningioma, chordoma, and chondrosarcoma. Reoperation for some malignant tumors is touched on briefly. This article does not cover vestibular schwannoma or paraganglioma.

Recurrent skull base tumors: general considerations

Diagnostic imaging studies

Most recurrent skull base tumors are asymptomatic at first; their early detection requires a high level of suspicion and routine periodic imaging

* Corresponding author.
E-mail address: anguyenh@stanford.edu (A. Nguyen-Huynh).

0030-6665/06/$ - see front matter © 2006 Elsevier Inc. All rights reserved.
doi:10.1016/j.otc.2006.04.006
oto.theclinics.com

studies of their former site. Usually, slow-growing benign tumors, such as low-grade meningioma and chondroid chordoma, are followed with annual imaging studies. More aggressive tumors, such as atypical meningioma or outright malignancies, should be followed radiographically every 6 months.

High-resolution, multiplanar MRI, with pre- and postgadolinium contrast and fat-saturation T1-weighted sequences, is the imaging study of choice to assess patients for recurrent skull base tumor [1]. To avoid misdiagnosis, it is essential to perform optimal imaging sequences. The resection bed often contains an abundance of enhancing tissue that requires a differential diagnosis among 1) recurrent tumor, 2) scar tissue, and 3) flaps and free tissue grafts placed during previous surgery. It is essential to use precontrast T1-weighted images and fat saturation techniques to reduce misinterpretation of signal from transplanted adipose tissue. Usually, scar can be discerned from tumor by its more linear pattern, but, ultimately, only serial images obtained to detect growth can exclude the presence of viable tumor definitively. In the case of an incomplete first resection, a postoperative scan should be obtained as soon as the patient is stable, to serve as a baseline for future comparison.

Radiotherapy leads to changes in the imaging characteristics of both the tumor and adjacent tissues [2]. The primary caveat is to not interpret early tumor swelling in the first 18 months after treatment as regrowth because it may represent transient radiation-induced edema in the process of tumor necrosis [3].

With any recurrent skull base lesion, a comprehensive understanding of the size and geometry of the lesion and its relationship to surrounding anatomy is essential. Specific attention should be paid to anatomic regions that may pose significant difficulty at the time of revision surgery. The presence of a tumor in the cavernous sinus, Meckel's cave, jugular foramen, or internal auditory canal (IAC) indicates the possibility of additional iatrogenic cranial neuropathy. Similarly, involvement of the carotid artery, the vertebrobasilar system, or dural sinuses should alert the surgeon to additional risk to the intracranial vasculature.

Additional bone imaging provided by CT can identify intraosseous tumor extension, common with chordoma and chondrosarcoma, and the formation of hyperostotic bone, commonly encountered with meningioma. This identification is useful to determine where particular attention may be needed at revision surgery. In addition, CT can demonstrate alterations in anatomic landmarks caused by disease or from a previous procedure.

Decision making in the management of recurrent tumors

The presence of a residual or recurrent tumor in the skull base after primary treatment presents a challenge to the neurotologic surgeon. These tumors tend to be more biologically aggressive and are located in more difficult-to-reach areas. As with primary disease, the options of watchful waiting, surgery, and radiotherapy must be considered carefully. A multidisciplinary team familiar with the management of these tumors is needed for optimal care. The recommended approach takes into account patient-related, tumor-related, and treatment-related factors.

Patient-related factors may be assessed by way of a thorough history and physical examination. Treatment may not be needed if it is unlikely that the tumor will cause significant morbidity over the patient's expected lifetime. The patient's age and comorbidities play a significant role in electing to forego revision surgery. The patient's functional status and any existing cranial neuropathy need to be evaluated carefully.

A number of tumor-related factors influence the approach to recurrent lesions. The expected growth rate can be estimated from histologic studies, warranting a diligent review of pathology specimens from the primary procedure. A lesion's expected biologic aggression can be inferred from the speed at which clinical symptoms manifest. Those causing more rapid morbidity are more likely to require revision surgery. Therefore, it is critical to distinguish benign from malignant disease.

Treatment-related factors include a critical appraisal of how much was attempted and accomplished during the previous resection. As a rule, if the initial resection was minimal, the tumor planes with adjacent neural and vascular structures may remain well defined, which would facilitate revision surgery. However, if a diligent attempt was undertaken initially to dissect tumor off surrounding structures, postsurgical scarring may make further dissection difficult. Similarly, the surgeon must consider which approach was used initially, and whether an alternative method may yield better exposure to problematic regions. In any case, surgeons considering revision surgery for skull base lesions need to appreciate the technical challenges inherent in such cases.

Effects of prior treatment on reoperation

The technical difficulties posed by reoperation in the posterior fossa are highly variable, possibly in part because of different degrees of meningeal inflammation caused by the initial procedure. With widespread inflammation, the arachnoid is diffusely tenacious and opalescent, which complicates the establishment of microdissection planes and may hinder the identification of vital structures.

As a general principle, it is usually advantageous to approach recurrent pathology by way of a new surgical route. Such a strategy tends to avoid scar and takes advantage of fresh tissue planes, and often provides access to regions left untreated during previous surgeries. For example, if a tumor has recurred after a retrosigmoid approach, the authors tend to select a transtemporal path in revision (and vice versa). Reopening a transtemporal craniotomy in the presence of dural contraction and thickening may provide only limited exposure.

In cases of planned subtotal tumor removal with possible reoperation, the authors prefer not to initiate and then abandon the dissection of a neural plane. Reoperation of a previously undissected tumor-nerve interface is typically much more effective than attempting to re-establish a partially developed plane in the face of adhesive scar tissue.

Prior surgery or tumor regrowth can alter normal vasculature, including the dural sinuses. If such a potential compromise is not taken into account, subsequent manipulation by cautery or retraction could result in venous congestion. Similarly, arterial blood supply may be tenuous after a previous surgery. The patency of arterial and venous channels can be evaluated preoperatively with magnetic resonance angiography or intravascular angiography.

Previous surgical attempts may have resulted in absent or obscured anatomic landmarks, so the surgeon doing the revision surgery may find far fewer of the customary reference points. Image-guided navigation techniques may help [4–7].

Neural injury is more possible in revision surgery because of scarring, especially in previously dissected areas, and also, to a lesser degree, because of thickening of the arachnoid and greater adhesiveness of planes in the vicinity of the prior surgery. The presence of encephalomalacia from prior retraction of the temporal lobe, cerebellum, or brainstem may render these structures more susceptible to injury from further surgery. Neurophysiologic monitoring is therefore highly recommended during revision surgery. Facial nerve monitoring is routine in most cases. Lower cranial nerve monitoring is indicated when the tumor extends to the jugular foramen level. Monitoring of trigeminal and extraocular motor nerves is indicated when the tumor extends to the Meckel's cave and the cavernous sinus. Monitoring of auditory brainstem evoked responses may help preserve hearing.

Reconstructive efforts can be challenging in revision surgery. The lack of local tissues suitable for reconstruction may lead to the development of cerebrospinal fluid (CFS) leak or pseudomeningocele formation.

Revision surgery may require resection of the tumor in direct contact with the paranasal sinuses or aerodigestive tract, which may bring a risk of contamination to the intracranial surgical field. In such situations, the resection should be staged to maintain a boundary between the normally contaminated mucosal surfaces and intracranial contents.

The effects of previous radiotherapy on the surgical field bring another set of challenges. It is most surgeons' experience that wide field radiation to the skull base increases the risk of wound healing problems and CSF leak, especially transcutaneous CSF leak [8]. Prior radiation also makes the brain more vulnerable to retraction, impairs the cranial nerve's ability to recuperate after operative manipulation, and makes vessels more prone to thrombosis. It also thickens the pia-arachnoid tumor interface, obscures dissection planes, and contributes to a greater risk of neural injury. As a general rule, increased reoperative risks after stereotactic radiotherapy (SRT) are more localized than those following wide beam therapy. Wound healing and CSF leak are less problematic after SRT than the fragility of structures in the confined radiation field.

Radiotherapy for recurrent skull base tumors

For malignant skull base lesions, either conventional or postoperative SRT is used routinely to try to control residual disease. Radiotherapy is also an alternative to surgery for patients who are poor surgical candidates for medical reasons, and for those with limited life expectancy.

SRT has an advantage over conventional therapy in that it can be highly conformal to the tumor. Using either a cobalt source (such as the Gamma knife) or a linear accelerator (as used in the Cyber knife), a large dose of energy can be delivered to the target while minimizing damage to the surrounding normal tissue. SRT has largely replaced brachytherapy and can be performed even after microsurgery and conventional radiotherapy have failed. Because of its highly conformal nature, SRT is also suitable for patients with recurrent benign tumors. In such cases, SRT may be offered as an alternative to revision surgery or as postoperative adjuvant therapy, enabling a more conservative resection. The best candidates for SRT are small, sharply demarcated tumors.

Radiotherapy of any type is contraindicated for large tumors with significant brainstem compression or edema. In such cases, radiotherapy may worsen compression and brain injury significantly as a result of post-treatment tumor edema. Radiotherapy for benign tumors in young patients needs to be approached with particular caution, given the potential for radiation-induced malignancy.

Meningioma

Meningioma is the second most common tumor found in the cerebellopontine angle (CPA) and IAC, accounting for about 10% of lesions in this area; most of the remaining tumors are vestibular schwannoma [9].

Meningioma originates from cap cells in arachnoid villi, finger-like invaginations of arachnoid tissue that project into dural veins and sinuses and provide the interface for absorption of CSF into the venous circulation. Arachnoid villi can also protrude through dura lining to penetrate the inner table of the calvarium [9]. Because they originate from the arachnoid, skull base meningiomas are often located in relatively inaccessible recesses between the brain and adjacent structures, rendering them difficult to fully resect and prone to recurrence.

Patterns of growth and classification

Meningiomas characteristically infiltrate adjacent dura, venous sinuses, and bone. They have two patterns of growth: globular and en-plaque.

Globular tumors are well circumscribed and tend to displace adjacent brain and nerves, while leaving the pia intact. En-plaque lesions are flat, more invasive into bone, and more likely to elicit hyperostosis. Tumor infiltration into bone does not necessarily indicate malignancy, however, because most meningiomas are histologically benign, and grow quite slowly, causing clinical symptoms by progressive local compression. The en-plaque form of meningioma is often difficult to resect completely, but may not require surgery as often because it is less likely than the globular form to generate significant mass effect. A meningioma can have both en-plaque and globular components, and its surgical resection can be tailored to address the component responsible for the clinical symptoms.

The World Health Organization (WHO) classifies meningiomas into three grades, based on histologic features and predicted behaviors (Table 1) [10,11]. The Grade I classification encompasses the most clinically benign subtypes and has the lowest risk of recurrence. Grade II includes clear-cell and chordoid subtypes and atypical meningiomas because they exhibit a similar increased risk of recurrence. Grade III consists of rhabdoid, papillary, and anaplastic meningiomas and has the highest risk of recurrence. Metastasis occurs in less than 0.1% of meningiomas and tends to seed the lungs, liver, and lymph nodes [12]. Papillary meningiomas, however, have a 55% chance of recurrence and a 20% chance of metastasis, illustrating the aggressive behavior of Grade III meningiomas [13].

Histologic classification is a significant predictor of recurrence and need for revision surgery. Recurrence rates of 3%, 38%, and 78% were reported for WHO Grades I, II, and III, respectively, after 5 years [14]. An elevated proliferation index and evidence of brain invasion are additional independent prognostic factors indicating high risk of recurrence above the WHO grade indicator [15,16].

Primary treatment and recurrence

Once diagnosed, meningiomas are usually treated surgically. Complete resection is usually the goal; however, this is not always possible because of the risk to surrounding vital structures, particularly in the case of

Table 1
WHO classification of meningiomas[a]

Classification	Histologic subtypes	Recurrence/ aggressiveness
Grade I	Meningoepithelial, fibrous, transitional, psammomatous, angiomatous, microcystic, secretory, lymphoplasmacyte-rich, and metaplastic	Low
Grade II	Atypical, clear-cell, and chordoid	Moderate
Grade III	Rhabdoid, papillary, and anaplastic	High

[a] High proliferation index and brain invasion are independent prognostic factors indicating increased risks for recurrence and aggressiveness for any given grade.

petroclival meningiomas that extend into the cavernous sinus or become densely adherent to the ventral brainstem (Fig. 1). Even when gross total resection is achieved, extensions of tumor infiltrating adjacent bone or dura may be missed.

Location of the tumor influences the possible extent of tumor removal. Complete excision of CPA meningiomas is accomplished in approximately 70% to 85% of cases [17–20]. Among meningiomas involving the posterior fossa, petroclival tumors have the worst prognosis for total removal, with Simpson Grades I and II (see later discussion) being achieved in only 25% to 47% of cases [21,22].

The extent of tumor removal at primary resection influences the likelihood of revision surgery being required in the future. The degree of resection has been classified according to Simpson's grading scheme (Table 2) [23]. Grade I is complete resection of the tumor together with its dural and bony attachments. Grade II is complete resection of the tumor with coagulation of its dural margin. Grade III is complete resection of the tumor without coagulation or removal of its dural margin. Grade IV is subtotal resection leaving residual tumor in situ. Grade V is simple decompression.

As expected, recurrence rates increase with time. At long-term follow-up, up to one third of patients will have a documented recurrence, despite apparent total tumor removal at the time of the primary procedure [24–26]. Recurrence rates after gross total resection have been documented to be 7% after 5 years, 20% after 10 years, and 32% after 15 years [25]. Progressive growth after subtotal removal is much higher, with rates found to be 37% after 5 years, 55% after 10 years, and 91% after 15 years [25].

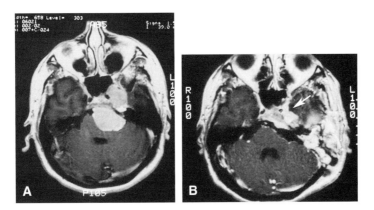

Fig. 1. (A) Axial T1-weighted postgadolinium MRI of a petroclival meningioma with extension into Meckel's cave. (B) Axial T1-weighted postgadolinium MRI of the tumor in A after subtotal resection, leaving a thin remnant of meningioma on the lateral aspect of the cavernous sinus (arrow). Incomplete resection was elected to avoid ophthalmoplegia because of the high risk of injury to cranial nerves III, IV, and VI associated with the radical resection of meningioma that has infiltrated the cavernous sinus.

Table 2
Simpson's grading of tumor removal and risks of recurrence

Classification	Extent of removal	Recurrence
Grade I	Complete resection including a dural margin and removal of any involved underlying bone	Low
Grade II	Complete resection with coagulation of dural attachment	Low
Grade III	Complete resection without a dural margin or coagulation of dural attachment	Moderate
Grade IV	Partial resection leaving residual tumor in situ	High
Grade V	Simple decompression	High

Follow-up protocol

The high rate of postoperative recurrence of meningioma even after apparent total removal necessitates long-term vigilance. Evidence of asymptomatic tumor regrowth should be monitored on serial imaging studies. Patients with incomplete resection need a postoperative MRI when medically stable to establish a baseline for future comparison. WHO Grade I tumors are the lowest risk and can be followed up with annual MRI. WHO Grades II and III tumors harbor the possibility of aggressive tumor regrowth. Therefore, postoperative radiotherapy is recommended highly, even if there is presumed complete resection. In addition, patients with WHO Grade II and III tumors need follow-up MRI every 6 months. After several years without demonstrable tumor regrowth, the interval between visits and imaging for all patients may be lengthened. High-risk patients likely need follow-up for the rest of their lives

Revision surgery

Often, the revision procedure can benefit from a different surgical approach that yields better exposure of problematic areas. The selection of an alternate approach has the added benefit of avoiding dissection in a previously operated field. If the primary surgery uses a retrosigmoid approach and there is no longer useful hearing, the translabyrinthine or transcochlear approach can provide excellent direct exposure. If hearing is to be preserved, a combined retrolabyrinthine/middle fossa approach can be used for tumor extending superiorly and anteriorly from the posterior fossa (Fig. 2). The far lateral approach can be used for tumors that extend inferiorly toward the foramen magnum.

Preoperative angiography can facilitate revision surgery for skull base meningioma. An angiogram can demonstrate the patency of involved dural sinuses and the adequacy of collateral venous drainage. Angiography with selective embolization of the tumor's arterial supply can reduce intraoperative blood loss substantially and facilitate orderly tumor microdissection [27]. As the tumor undergoes necrosis from embolization, it also softens and becomes more amenable to removal by an ultrasonic suction aspirator

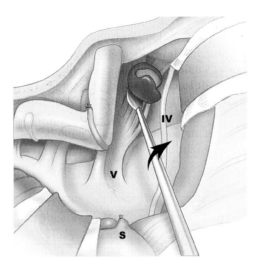

Fig. 2. Combined retrolabyrinthine-subtemporal approach to the Meckel's cave portion of a petroclival meningioma. The sigmoid sinus (S) is retracted posteriorly. The dura and the tentorium have been opened. The cranial nerves IV and V are labeled.

[9]. Angiography for meningiomas carries the known risks of stroke and intracranial hemorrhage, however, which must be weighed against its potential benefits [28].

Meningiomas tend to occur near major dural sinuses. When involved with recurrent tumor, these should be resected if possible. The vein of Labbé should be preserved because it might be the sole outflow tract for the temporal lobe. This vein has a variable course and often enters the transverse sinus posterior to the transverse-sigmoid sinus junction, but can sometimes enter into the superior petrosal sinus. Loss of this vein can cause a venous infarct, resulting in serious speech and memory disturbances, and seizures, especially if the dominant side is affected [29].

Because viable meningioma remnants may reside in underlying hyperostotic bone, it is important to drill away this abnormal bone during radical tumor removal [30]. Meningiomas frequently possess an adjacent "dural tail" on MRI. Histologically, this is usually peritumoral hypervascularity without neoplastic cells, and thus is not likely a case of recurrence following resection [31]. However, it has been observed in SRT that patients treated with less conformal plans, which better cover the dural tail, have improved tumor control rates [32].

The trend in skull base meningioma management has been to undertake less than complete resection when radical resection would compromise functionally important neural structures or risk vital arteries. The recent availability of SRT has improved the viability of this practice. [33]. This modality is an attractive option for halting growth in tumor remnants and thus avoiding the higher morbidity of radical operation.

Chordoma

Chordoma is a neoplasm that originates from ectodermal remnants of the notochord, the rod-shaped embryonic structure that defines the longitudinal axis. Because of its embryonic origin, chordoma occurs in the axial skeleton from the base of the skull to the coccyx. Skull base chordomas comprise about one third of all chordomas, and most involve the clivus. Chordoma is a very rare tumor with an incidence of 0.08 per 100,000 in the United States [34].

Chordoma is a histologically benign, slow-growing, yet relentless neoplasm, which makes revision surgery a consideration during its management. It infiltrates along the lines of least resistance, both within and adjacent to bone. A clival chordoma can extend anteriorly to the anterior and middle cranial fossae, orbit, paranasal sinuses, and nasopharynx; laterally to the petrous apex and cavernous sinus; inferiorly to the infratemporal fossa; or posteriorly to involve the CPA in the posterior cranial fossa. Even though most chordomas remain extradural, these tumors can occasionally transgress dura.

MRI is the primary diagnostic approach, showing chordoma to be isointense on T1-weighted images, with bright gadolinium enhancement, and hyperintense on T2-weighted images. High-resolution CT can demonstrate the extent of bone destruction and the involvement of any neural foramina. Intratumoral calcification is common. Both modalities are essential to ascertain the most efficient surgical approach to the lesion. MRI is the most useful imaging technique for postoperative follow-up.

Primary treatment and recurrence

Surgery is the mainstay of treatment for chordoma, but complete resection is achieved rarely. Total removal of clival chordomas is limited by the tumor's tendency to infiltrate into inaccessible regions, and its intimate relationship with vital structures, such as the vertebrobasilar system, lower cranial nerves, and brainstem. The tumors can also involve the pituitary gland, the optic chiasm, and other cranial nerves. The absence of a capsule, the gelatinous nature of the tumor, and the possibility of seeding the surgical bed also make complete resection difficult. Clival chordoma has been found to recur along previous surgical pathways [35].

In a review of 128 cases of microscopically confirmed skull base chordomas in the United States between 1973 and 1995, the median survival was 6.9 years, with 5- and 10-year relative survival rates of 65% and 47%, respectively [34]. Relative survival rate was defined as the ratio of observed survival over expected survival, based on age, sex and race.

The current standard of treatment is maximum surgical resection followed by conformal photon or proton radiotherapy. Two hundred and four subjects with skull base or cervical chordomas treated with surgery and proton radiation therapy to 70 Gy showed a recurrence rate of 29%

at a mean follow-up of 54 months [36]. Among the treatment failures, 95% had local recurrence, 5% had surgical pathway recurrence, 3% developed regional lymph node metastases, and 20% had distant metastases. Lungs and bones were the most common sites of dissemination. Salvage surgery was performed in 49 subjects, with only three apparently complete resections. In 14% of the salvaged cases, symptoms were either stable or improved and there was no evidence of disease progression. Overall, the 2- and 5-year actuarial survival rates after the first recurrence were 63% and 6%, respectively.

Gross total resection at primary surgery gives the best chance for cure. In a study of 42 subjects with skull base chordoma, the eight patients who had complete or near-total resection enjoyed 100% 5-year survival without evidence of tumor regrowth [37]. The remaining 34 subjects who did not have complete or near total resection at their first surgeries required postoperative radiation to 50–65 Gy and 22 additional operations to achieve a 65% 5-year survival rate [37]. Operative mortality was 0% with primary surgery and 4% with revision surgery. The rate of postoperative CSF leak was about 17% for both groups.

Skull base chordomas are among the most difficult tumors to cure even with combined therapy, but repeat operations can often relieve symptoms and extend life [38].

Follow-up protocol

Even though chordoma is histologically benign, it is a biologically aggressive tumor. Its follow-up protocol is similar to that of high-risk meningiomas, as discussed previously. Consideration of postoperative SRT is highly recommended, and patients need follow-up imaging with serial MRI every 6 months.

Revision surgery

Most primary chordomas confined to the midline region of the clivus are resected by way of a ventral extradural (eg, transoral or trans-sphenoethmoidal) approach. Recurrence tends to occur when the tumor has spread either intradurally in front of the midbrain or pons, or laterally through intraosseous growth to a position behind the intrapetrous carotid artery. Such recurrences are not accessible with an anterior approach; a lateral exposure is necessary. The authors' favored approach in such cases is a combined middle and posterior fossa craniotomy, achieved through a limited petrosectomy (Fig. 3) [39]. In some cases, particularly those of recurrences that extended laterally, an infratemporal fossa approach combined with a transpetrosal or far-lateral approach can be used [37]. Image-guided surgical navigation and endoscopic techniques are useful adjunctive measures for obtaining the best possible degree of resection [4–7].

Chordoma is resistant to conventional radiation therapy with high-energy photons in the range of 50–55 Gy [40]. Higher doses of photon

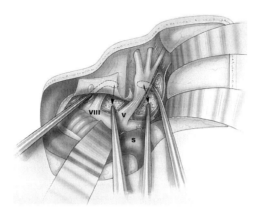

Fig. 3. Lateral approach (combined retrolabyrinthine-subtemporal) to an extensive clival chordoma with a major intracranial component having recurred after an incomplete anterior resection. The sigmoid sinus (S) is retracted posteriorly, and the dura has been opened. Cranial
nerves V and VIII are visible. Arrows point to tumor being removed by a combination of suction and blunt dissection. (*From* Blevins NH, Jackler RK, Kaplan MJ, et al. Combined transpetrosal-subtemporal craniotomy for clival tumors with extension into the posterior fossa.
Laryngoscope 1995;105(9 Pt 1):975–82; with permission.)

radiation cannot be delivered safely in a conventional manner because they
exceed the tolerance of the brainstem [41]. To deliver higher energy with
more precision, proton beam radiation can be used. The intensity of a proton
beam can be modulated precisely along its path with a sharp fall-off within
a few millimeters of its Bragg peak. Proton beam radiotherapy is the most
effective form of radiotherapy against chordoma, but it is very expensive
and available at very few centers [42]. Early results of SRT for chordoma
are promising, but not yet as good as those obtained with proton beam
treatment [43–45].

Chondrosarcoma

Chondrosarcoma is a rare, slow-growing cartilage malignancy. Skull base
chondrosarcoma characteristically arises from the foramen lacerum at the
petroclival synchondrosis [46–48]. By infiltrating bone or following the crevices that interconnect the intra- and extracranial spaces, a petroclival chondrosarcoma can extend posteriorly to the CPA; laterally to the IAC;
inferiorly to the jugular fossa; superiorly to the parasellar region; and anteriorly into the sphenoid sinus. The tumor easily invades Dorello's canal,
causing abducens palsy.

Chordoma and chondrosarcoma are different tumors, but they are often
considered together because they both occur in the central skull base and
have nearly identical radiographic appearance. Both tumors are isointense
on T1-weighted MRI, with bright gadolinium enhancement, and hyperintense on T2-weighted MRI. Intratumoral calcification is common in both

tumors, as seen on CT scans [49]. The location of the lesions is a major factor in differentiating chordoma from chondrosarcoma. Chordoma is almost exclusively a midline lesion, whereas chondrosarcoma is located off midline in the petroclival junction.

As with chordoma, high-resolution CT can demonstrate the extent of bone destruction and the involvement of any neural foramina by chondrosarcoma. Both CT and MRI are essential in determining the most efficient surgical approach to the lesion. MRI is the most useful imaging technique for postoperative follow-up.

Primary treatment and recurrence

The current standard of primary treatment for chondrosarcoma is combined surgery and postoperative radiation. When treated with surgery alone, the recurrence rate of chondrosarcoma is 53%, with a mean time to recurrence of 32 months [50]. Oghalai and colleagues [48] found that lack of postoperative radiation correlated significantly with an increased risk of recurrence (odds ratio, 28; $P = .007$). Near total resection, leaving a small, well-cauterized remnant of tumor to preserve the internal carotid artery or other vital structure, was not associated with increased risk of recurrence [48]. Subtotal resection, leaving a remnant visible in postoperative MRI, however, was associated with an increased risk of recurrence.

In a study of 200 subjects with chondrosarcoma treated with surgery and proton therapy in the range of 64–80 Gy and followed for a mean of 65 months, the 5- and 10-year local control rates were 99% and 98%, respectively, and the 5- and 10-year disease-specific survival rates were both 99% [51]. Similar studies of combined surgery and proton therapy reported 5-year survival rates of 83% to 94% and 5-year local control rates of 78% to 91% [48,50]. These results show that the prognosis for chondrosarcoma is much better than that of chordoma. Early results of SRT for chordoma are promising, but not yet as good as those of proton beam treatment [43–45].

Follow-up protocol

Even though chondrosarcoma responds well to combined surgery and postoperative radiation, it is still a malignant tumor, and patients need follow up-imaging with annual MRI.

Revision surgery

Petroclival chondrosarcoma often wraps around the medial surface of the intrapetrous carotid artery. Neither a subtemporal nor a transtemporal approach easily exposes a tumor component situated beneath the horizontal course of the intrapetrous carotid artery, making this a likely area of persistent or recurrent disease. If imaging studies before revision surgery confirm the presence of a tumor in this area, it can be exposed through an infratemporal fossa approach (Fig. 4) [48,52].

Recurrent disease can be treated with further surgical resection or SRT as needed, although recurrence is still associated with a worse prognosis [53]. Systemic chemotherapy may be beneficial to some patients with multiply recurrent disease [54].

Reoperation in malignant skull base lesions

In general, results following major cranial base resection for high-grade malignant tumors (eg, squamous cell carcinoma, adenocystic carcinoma) have been disappointing. As a general rule, recurrence after prior resection and radiation therapy is not amenable to repeat resection. Some have advocated superaggressive salvage surgery, including carotid resection and even vascular bypass, but the possibility of a cure in such cases is remote and the risk of morbidity is high. Even when the vascular anatomy appears favorable and the patient passes a balloon occlusion test, a significant risk of stroke still exists [55,56].

Pediatric sarcoma (eg, rhabdomyosarcoma) involving the cranial base often requires a biopsy, followed by chemotherapy. Because of the higher risk

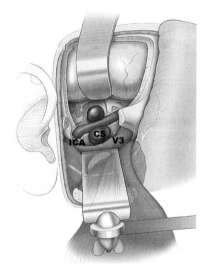

Fig. 4. Recommended anterior subtemporal-infratemporal fossa approach to an extensive petroclival chondrosarcoma. When approached using a purely lateral (transtemporal) or superior (subtemporal) technique, the portion of the chondrosarcoma (CS) lying inferior to the intrapetrous segment of the internal carotid artery (ICA) may be difficult to exenterate completely and can lead to recurrence. (*From* Oghalai JS, Buxbaum JL, Jackler RK, et al. Skull base chondrosarcoma originating from the petroclival junction. Otol Neurotol 2005;26(5):1052–60; with permission.)

of treatment failure in parameningeal foci, a second and more definitive resection is sometimes recommended. The goal is cytoreduction, rather than radical resection, to facilitate the effectiveness of chemotherapy [57].

Summary

Because the skull base is an anatomically complex structure, skull base tumors can hide easily in the crevices that interconnect the intra- and extracranial spaces and intermingle with important neurovascular structures. Often, total surgical resection of these tumors is not possible, and even with postoperative adjuvant radiotherapy, some recurrences after treatment are inevitable. Early detection of recurrent skull base tumors requires clinical vigilance and periodic imaging studies. The management of recurrent skull base tumors presents many challenges beyond those associated with primary procedures. A multidisciplinary setting that includes modern microsurgery and SRT provides patients with optimal care.

References

[1] Wallace RC, Dean BL, Beals SP, et al. Post treatment imaging of the skull base. Semin Ultrasound CT MR 2003;24(3):164–81.

[2] Plowman PN. Stereotactic radiosurgery VIII. The classification of post radiation reactions. Br J Neurosurg 1999;13(3):256–64.

[3] Chang JH, Chang JW, Choi JY, et al. Complications after gamma knife radiosurgery for benign meningiomas. J Neurol Neurosurg Psychiatry 2003;74(2):226–30.

[4] Hassfeld S, Zoller J, Albert FK, et al. Preoperative planning and intraoperative navigation in skull base surgery. J Craniomaxillofac Surg 1998;26(4):220–5.

[5] Kurtsoy A, Menku A, Tucer B, et al. Neuronavigation in skull base tumors. Minim Invasive Neurosurg 2005;48(1):7–12.

[6] Schul C, Wassmann H, Skopp GB, et al. Surgical management of intraosseous skull base tumors with aid of operating arm system. Comput Aided Surg 1998;3(6):312–9.

[7] Sure U, Alberti O, Petermeyer M, et al. Advanced image-guided skull base surgery. Surg Neurol 2000;53(6):563–72 [discussion: 572].

[8] Nishioka H, Haraoka J, Ikeda Y. Risk factors of cerebrospinal fluid rhinorrhea following transsphenoidal surgery. Acta Neurochir (Wien) 2005;147(11):1163–6.

[9] Irving RM. Meningiomas of the internal auditory canal and cerebellopontine angle. In: Jackler RK, Driscoll CLW, editors. Tumors of the ear and temporal bone. Philadelphia: Lippincott Williams & Wilkins; 2000. p. 219–35.

[10] Kleihues P, Louis DN, Scheithauer BW, et al. The WHO classification of tumors of the nervous system. J Neuropathol Exp Neurol 2002;61(3):215–25 [discussion: 226–9].

[11] Kleihues P, Sobin LH. World Health Organization classification of tumors. Cancer 2000; 88(12):2887.

[12] Kepes JJ. Meningiomas: biology, pathology, and differential diagnosis. New York: Masson Publishing USA, Inc; 1982. p. 112–23.

[13] Pasquier B, Gasnier F, Pasquier D, et al. Papillary meningioma. Clinicopathologic study of seven cases and review of the literature. Cancer 1986;58(2):299–305.

[14] Kallio M, Sankila R, Hakulinen T, et al. Factors affecting operative and excess long-term mortality in 935 patients with intracranial meningioma. Neurosurgery 1992;31(1): 2–12.

[15] Perry A, Scheithauer BW, Stafford SL, et al. "Malignancy" in meningiomas: a clinicopath-
    ologic study of 116 patients, with grading implications. Cancer 1999;85(9):2046–56.
[16] Perry A, Stafford SL, Scheithauer BW, et al. Meningioma grading: an analysis of histologic
    parameters. Am J Surg Pathol 1997;21(12):1455–65.
[17] Samii M, Ammirati M, Mahran A, et al. Surgery of petroclival meningiomas: report of 24
    cases. Neurosurgery 1989;24(1):12–7.
[18] Arriaga M, Shelton C, Nassif P, et al. Selection of surgical approaches for meningiomas af-
    fecting the temporal bone. Otolaryngol Head Neck Surg 1992;107(6 Pt 1):738–44.
[19] Bricolo AP, Turazzi S, Talacchi A, et al. Microsurgical removal of petroclival meningiomas:
    a report of 33 patients. Neurosurgery 1992;31(5):813–28 [discussion: 828].
[20] Schaller B, Heilbronner R, Pfaltz CR, et al. Preoperative and postoperative auditory and fa-
    cial nerve function in cerebellopontine angle meningiomas. Otolaryngol Head Neck Surg
    1995;112(2):228–34.
[21] Thomas NW, King TT. Meningiomas of the cerebellopontine angle. A report of 41 cases. Br
    J Neurosurg 1996;10(1):59–68.
[22] Mayberg MR, Symon L. Meningiomas of the clivus and apical petrous bone. Report of 35
    cases. J Neurosurg 1986;65(2):160–7.
[23] Simpson D. The recurrence of intracranial meningiomas after surgical treatment. J Neurol
    Neurosurg Psychiatry 1957;20(1):22–39.
[24] Adegbite AB, Khan MI, Paine KW, et al. The recurrence of intracranial meningiomas after
    surgical treatment. J Neurosurg 1983;58(1):51–6.
[25] Mirimanoff RO, Dosoretz DE, Linggood RM, et al. Meningioma: analysis of recurrence and
    progression following neurosurgical resection. J Neurosurg 1985;62(1):18–24.
[26] Jaaskelainen J. Seemingly complete removal of histologically benign intracranial meningi-
    oma: late recurrence rate and factors predicting recurrence in 657 patients. A multivariate
    analysis. Surg Neurol 1986;26(5):461–9.
[27] Dean BL, Flom RA, Wallace RC, et al. Efficacy of endovascular treatment of meningiomas:
    evaluation with matched samples. AJNR Am J Neuroradiol 1994;15(9):1675–80.
[28] Kallmes DF, Evans AJ, Kaptain GJ, et al. Hemorrhagic complications in embolization of
    a meningioma: case report and review of the literature. Neuroradiology 1997;39(12):871–80.
[29] Lustig LR, Jackler RK. The vulnerability of the vein of Labbé during combined craniot-
    omies of the posterior and middle fossae. Skull Base 1998;8:1–9.
[30] Pieper DR, Al-Mefty O, Hanada Y, et al. Hyperostosis associated with meningioma of the
    cranial base: secondary changes or tumor invasion. Neurosurgery 1999;44(4):742–6 [discus-
    sion: 746–7].
[31] Kawahara Y, Niiro M, Yokoyama S, et al. Dural congestion accompanying meningioma in-
    vasion into vessels: the dural tail sign. Neuroradiology 2001;43(6):462–5.
[32] DiBiase SJ, Kwok Y, Yovino S, et al. Factors predicting local tumor control after gamma
    knife stereotactic radiosurgery for benign intracranial meningiomas. Int J Radiat Oncol
    Biol Phys 2004;60(5):1515–9.
[33] Tonn JC. Microneurosurgery and radiosurgery–an attractive combination. Acta Neurochir
    Suppl (Wien) 2004;91:103–8.
[34] McMaster ML, Goldstein AM, Bromley CM, et al. Chordoma: incidence and survival pat-
    terns in the United States, 1973–1995. Cancer Causes Control 2001;12(1):1–11.
[35] Fischbein NJ, Kaplan MJ, Holliday RA, et al. Recurrence of clival chordoma along the sur-
    gical pathway. AJNR Am J Neuroradiol 2000;21(3):578–83.
[36] Fagundes MA, Hug EB, Liebsch NJ, et al. Radiation therapy for chordomas of the base of
    skull and cervical spine: patterns of failure and outcome after relapse. Int J Radiat Oncol Biol
    Phys 1995;33(3):579–84.
[37] Crockard HA, Steel T, Plowman N, et al. A multidisciplinary team approach to skull base
    chordomas. J Neurosurg 2001;95(2):175–83.
[38] Kyoshima K, Oikawa S, Kanaji M, et al. Repeat operations in the management of clival
    chordomas: palliative surgery. J Clin Neurosci 2003;10(5):571–8.

[39] Blevins NH, Jackler RK, Kaplan MJ, et al. Combined transpetrosal-subtemporal craniotomy for clival tumors with extension into the posterior fossa. Laryngoscope 1995;105(9 Pt 1): 975–82.

[40] Catton C, O'Sullivan B, Bell R, et al. Chordoma: long-term follow-up after radical photon irradiation. Radiother Oncol 1996;41(1):67–72.

[41] Debus J, Hug EB, Liebsch NJ, et al. Brainstem tolerance to conformal radiotherapy of skull base tumors. Int J Radiat Oncol Biol Phys 1997;39(5):967–75.

[42] Noel G, Feuvret L, Calugaru V, et al. Chordomas of the base of the skull and upper cervical spine. One hundred patients irradiated by a 3D conformal technique combining photon and proton beams. Acta Oncol 2005;44(7):700–8.

[43] Feigl GC, Bundschuh O, Gharabaghi A, et al. Evaluation of a new concept for the management of skull base chordomas and chondrosarcomas. J Neurosurg 2005;102(Suppl):165–70.

[44] Krishnan S, Foote RL, Brown PD, et al. Radiosurgery for cranial base chordomas and chondrosarcomas. Neurosurgery 2005;56(4):777–84 [discussion: 777–84].

[45] Muthukumar N, Kondziolka D, Lunsford LD, et al. Stereotactic radiosurgery for chordoma and chondrosarcoma: further experiences. Int J Radiat Oncol Biol Phys 1998;41(2):387–92.

[46] Coltrera MD, Googe PB, Harrist TJ, et al. Chondrosarcoma of the temporal bone. Diagnosis and treatment of 13 cases and review of the literature. Cancer 1986;58(12):2689–96.

[47] Lau DP, Wharton SB, Antoun NM, et al. Chondrosarcoma of the petrous apex. Dilemmas in diagnosis and treatment. J Laryngol Otol 1997;111(4):368–71.

[48] Oghalai JS, Buxbaum JL, Jackler RK, et al. Skull base chondrosarcoma originating from the petroclival junction. Otol Neurotol 2005;26(5):1052–60.

[49] Oot RF, Melville GE, New PF, et al. The role of MR and CT in evaluating clival chordomas and chondrosarcomas. AJR Am J Roentgenol 1988;151(3):567–75.

[50] Korten AG, ter Berg HJ, Spincemaille GH, et al. Intracranial chondrosarcoma: review of the literature and report of 15 cases. J Neurol Neurosurg Psychiatry 1998;65(1):88–92.

[51] Rosenberg AE, Nielsen GP, Keel SB, et al. Chondrosarcoma of the base of the skull: a clinicopathologic study of 200 cases with emphasis on its distinction from chordoma. Am J Surg Pathol 1999;23(11):1370–8.

[52] Kveton JF, Brackmann DE, Glasscock ME 3rd, et al. Chondrosarcoma of the skull base. Otolaryngol Head Neck Surg 1986;94(1):23–32.

[53] Kocher M, Voges J, Staar S, et al. Linear accelerator radiosurgery for recurrent malignant tumors of the skull base. Am J Clin Oncol 1998;21(1):18–22.

[54] La Rocca RV, Morgan KW, Paris K, et al. Recurrent chondrosarcoma of the cranial base: a durable response to ifosfamide-doxorubicin chemotherapy. J Neurooncol 1999;41(3): 281–3.

[55] Wolfe SQ, Tummala RP, Morcos JJ. Cerebral revascularization in skull base tumors. Skull Base 2005;15(1):71–82.

[56] Chazono H, Okamoto Y, Matsuzaki Z, et al. Carotid artery resection: preoperative temporary occlusion is not always an accurate predictor of collateral blood flow. Acta Otolaryngol 2005;125(2):196–200.

[57] Wharam MD Jr. Rhabdomyosarcoma of parameningeal sites. Semin Radiat Oncol 1997; 7(3):212–6 [r].

**ELSEVIER
SAUNDERS**

Otolaryngol Clin N Am
39 (2006) 801–813

OTOLARYNGOLOGIC
CLINICS
OF NORTH AMERICA

Revision BAHA Surgery

Robert A. Battista, MD, FACS[a,b,*],
Philip D. Littlefield, MD[a]

[a]*Northwestern University Feinberg School of Medicine, Chicago, IL, USA*
[b]*Ear Institute of Chicago, LLC, Hinsdale, IL, USA*

The osseointegrated auditory implant (BAHA) is a system used for hearing rehabilitation through direct bone conduction. As such, the BAHA is an alternative to traditional bone, air conduction, and contralateral routing of offside signal (CROS) hearing devices. The BAHA system consists of three components: a titanium implant, a percutaneous abutment, and a sound processor. The titanium implant is implanted surgically behind the hearing-impaired ear and is allowed to osseointegrate into the skull. The percutaneous abutment is then attached to the implant, and the sound processor snaps on to the abutment after an appropriate period of osseointegration. Unlike conventional bone conduction devices, the BAHA does not require pressure on the skin for coupling, and sound vibrations are not attenuated by skin and soft tissue. Instead, the BAHA vibrates the skull directly through the titanium implant. In addition, some of the problems of air-conduction devices (eg, chronic otorrhea, cerumen impaction) are avoided because the BAHA is not worn in the ear canal.

The BAHA has undergone many innovative changes since the first clinical trial of the system in 1977 in Sweden. These innovations, coupled with its widespread clinical use, have led to several clinical applications. In the United States, the BAHA has received Food and Drug Administration (FDA) clearance for use in adults and children (aged five and older) with unilateral or bilateral conductive or mixed hearing loss, or unilateral profound sensorineural hearing loss (SNHL), also known as single-sided deafness. In 2001, the FDA approved bilateral fittings for conductive or mixed hearing losses. The BAHA is manufactured and distributed by Bone Anchored Solutions, a Cochlear Group company.

* Corresponding author: Ear Institute of Chicago, LLC, 950 North York Road, Suite 102, Hinsdale, IL 60521.

E-mail address: r-battista2@northwestern.edu (R.A. Battista).

Box 1. Clinical indications for BAHA implantation

Conductive or mixed hearing loss
Patients with chronic otorrhea
- Chronic otitis externa
- Chronic otitis media

Patients with congenital aural atresia (microtia)
Patients with other conductive or mixed hearing loss
- Ossicular discontinuity/fixation in an only-hearing ear
- External canal closure from skull base procedure

Patients with air-conduction or conventional bone conduction
  hearing aids who desire a more comfortable fit using the BAHA

Unilateral, profound sensorineural hearing loss (single-sided deafness)

Numerous studies have shown that the BAHA is a safe and effective system for specific clinical (Box 1) and audiological (Box 2) situations. The device has two different sound processors: the Divino (Fig. 1), and the Cordelle. The Divino is an ear-level device and the Cordelle is a body-worn processor. The Cordelle provides approximately 13 decibels (dB) more gain than the Divino.

As with any surgical procedure, there are complications or traumatic events that may require revision surgery. The purpose of this article is to discuss indications for revision, and specific recommendations for revision surgical technique. In general, indications for revision BAHA surgery can be divided into (1) failure of fixture osseointegration; (2) bone overgrowth; or (3) skin reaction or skin loss. Some problems requiring revision can be prevented by proper surgical technique during the initial operation. For this reason, the article reviews some key surgical procedure points important

---

Box 2. Audiological criteria for BAHA candidacy

Conductive or mixed hearing loss
Degree of air–bone gap irrelevant
Pure tone average (0.5, 1, 2, 3 kHz) bone conduction ≤ 45 dB

Single-sided deafness
Profound SNHL in the impaired ear (pure tone average >90 dB
  and word recognition score <20%)
Normal hearing in the contralateral ear (pure tone average <20
  dB and word recognition score >80%)

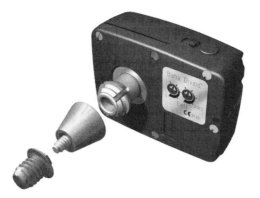

Fig. 1. The BAHA sound system. From left to right, the titanium fixture, the abutment, and the rear view of the Divino sound processor. (Courtesy of Cochlear Limited; with permission.)

for a successful operation. Full details of the surgical procedure have been published elsewhere [1].

Primary BAHA surgery overview

BAHA implantation is performed in either a one- or a two-stage procedure. The two-stage procedure is reserved for children under 18 years old and for patients with a previously irradiated temporal bone. In both the one- and two-stage procedures, the authors recommend a minimum of a 3-month period before loading the implant with the sound processor. This time period is necessary to allow for complete osseointegration.

When creating the skin flap, the authors recommend the use of Dermatome (made by Bone Anchored Solutions, a Cochlear Group company), designed specifically for BAHA surgery. The Dermatome creates a skin flap with a thickness of 0.6 mm. At this thickness, the surgeon is ensured of a depilated flap of sufficient depth for proper wound healing.

Throughout the surgical procedure, the surgeon must keep thermal and mechanical trauma to a minimum to ensure adequate osseointegration. Heat trauma can result in a local fibrous reaction, leading to poor osseointegration and implant failure. All debris must be removed from the hole before fixture insertion. Mastoid air cells decrease bone–titanium contact and should be avoided. The minimum recommended fixture depth is 3 mm because shorter lengths have a much greater chance for failure [2]. The titanium fixture should never come in contact with anything other than bone or dura.

The removal of surrounding subcutaneous tissue is a crucial step in BAHA implantation. Great care must be taken to reduce the soft tissue surrounding the implant, in a radius of approximately 1.25 cm. Removal of soft tissue helps to prevent postoperative prolapse of soft tissue onto the abutment and should result in an area of very thin, hairless skin around the abutment.

Finally, prior to securing the skin flap, the periosteum under the skin flap should be thinned to one layer thickness. There should be little to no tension on the skin flap when reapproximating the flap to the skin edges. Thinning the periosteum and creating a tension-free skin flap helps to prevent movement of the skin flap during healing. Movement of the flap may lead to inflammation and skin overgrowth.

Indications for revision BAHA surgery

Failure of osseointegration

Symptoms and signs of osseointegration failure can vary. In the most severe situation, the abutment–fixture complex may be so loose that it falls out. At other times, a fibrous attachment is present; the fixture remains in place but the patient experiences little or no sound, or complains of sound distortion when the sound processor is fitted. In these situations, the abutment–fixture complex will spin freely when an attempt is made to tighten the abutment in the office.

Several factors must be considered for adequate osseointegration. Proper surgical technique at the initial surgery is paramount. The thickness of the bone is also important. The thickness of the temporal bone is often a function of the patient's age at implantation and his/her craniofacial anatomy. Patients with craniofacial syndromes often have thin bone in the area of planned implantation. One reason for implant losses without any known trauma is idiopathic bone resorption at the bone–metal interface [3].

The current FDA guidelines recommend a lower age limit of five years for BAHA implantation. These guidelines are based on the finding that most children of five years or older have bone thickness adequate to hold a 3-mm fixture. Some centers, however, have reported implantation in children between the ages of 3 and 5 years, with good results [4–7]. Children as young as 1 year have been implanted successfully by way of a three-stage procedure that begins with bone grafting to the recipient site, or a two-stage procedure that includes bone augmentation during the first stage, with a period of more than 3 months between stages [8]. In general, fixture lengths of less than 3 mm have a much higher failure rate than longer fixtures [2,8,9].

If the thickest bone that can be found is 2.0 mm to 2.5 mm thick, then the surgeon has a few options for fixture placement. One option is to secure a fixture slightly longer than the depth of the bone (ie, a 2.5-mm fixture in 2.0-mm–thick bone; a 3.0-mm fixture in 2.5-mm–thick bone). In this situation, a 4-month or greater, rather than a 3-month, period of osseointegration is recommended before loading the implant. Some investigators have reported success with this technique [5,7–9].

Another option when the bone is thin is to close the wound, and return 6 to 12 months later when the temporal bone is thicker. A final option consists of bone augmentation performed in a two-stage procedure. In the first stage, a 3-mm fixture can be used with 1 mm of the fixture exposed above the skull. Bone chips and dust can be packed under the flange of the fixture, and a Gortex or expanded polytetrafluoroethylene (e-PTFE) membrane can be placed over the fixture to secure the area (Fig. 2) [3,10]. Again, a 4-month or greater, rather than a 3-month, period of osseointegration is recommended before loading the implant.

Previous radiation also has a negative effect on osseointegration. Implant failure is much higher in radiated bone and is believed to occur from localized osteoradionecrosis [11]. Adjuvant hyperbaric oxygen with BAHA insertion, however, will improve the chance for success considerably [12].

In some cases, a loosely fitted fixture at the time of primary surgery may result in failure of osseointegration. The chance for osseointegration is increased if the implant is loaded 4 or more months after implantation [7].

Trauma is another reason for fixture loss. Although trauma can occur at any age, it is far more common in the pediatric population.

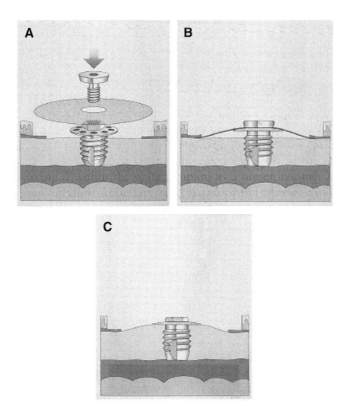

Fig. 2. (A) The fixture with the e-PTFE membrane before it is put in place. (B) The e-PTFE membrane on top of the fixture, with the edges of the membrane underneath the periosteum. The space around the flange of the fixture accommodates bone growth. (C) At the second stage, the space has been filled with bone to support the fixture. (Courtesy of Anders Tjellström, MD, PhD.)

Many authors recommend "banking" a second "sleeper" fixture during implant surgery in populations with relatively high failure rates (ie, pediatric patients, those with craniofacial disorder, and previously irradiated patients) [7,9,10], to allow a spare to osseointegrate should the primary fixture fail.

Bone overgrowth

The possibility of bone overgrowth should be considered when a loose abutment cannot be tightened. Bone overgrowth is found exclusively in children, especially between the ages of 5 and 11 [5,8]. Bone growth during this time period is significant, with the growth of the temporal and parietal bones being appositional (ie, lamellar). Because growth is appositional, bone overgrowth can occur while the implant position does not change in the sagittal direction.

Skin reaction

Skin reactions are divided into two types: local wound inflammation or infection, and skin overgrowth. Local wound inflammation around the abutment is commonly classified according to the clinical scoring system of Holgers and colleagues [13], as follows: 0 = no irritation; 1 = slight redness; 2 = red and moist; 3 = same as 2, but also with granulation tissue formed; and 4 = skin irritation of such a degree that the abutment has to be removed. Treatment of the skin reaction may vary, depending on its grade (Anders Tjellstrom, personal communication, 2006). For Grade 1 reactions, local antibiotic ointment is recommended. Reapplying the healing cap, and wrapping the area with antibiotic gauze for a period of time, may treat Grade 2 reactions. Grade 3 and 4 reactions require revision surgery, as outlined in the Revision BAHA surgery section.

Inflammation around the abutment is, in general, more common in children than in adults [4,9,14–19]. The overall rate of skin reaction around the implant ranges from 7.1% to 39.6%; the reactions vary in severity from reddish discoloration to loss of the fixture [12–14,20,21]. Persistent, chronic infections around the implant may be due to Staphylococcus aureus [21]. More severe infections can also occur, ranging from osteomyelitis with loss of the fixture, to intracerebral abscess [22,23]. Of the two reported cases of intracerebral abscess, one case occurred in an adult who developed osteomyelitis after an abutment replacement 8 years after initial surgery [22]. The second case was in a child who developed an intracerebral abscess several weeks after showing signs of significant improvement when being treated for a skin infection. Neither report clarified whether dura was exposed at the time of the original surgery. With these cases in mind, it is recommended that a CT or MRI be performed in the case of neurologic symptoms or therapy-resistant headaches, or if local evidence of infection persists after placement of a BAHA sound processor.

The other form of skin reaction is skin overgrowth, a frequent problem after BAHA implantation, that may engulf the abutment partially, near totally (Fig. 3), or completely. This problem can occur at any time after implantation. In general, skin overgrowth occurs more frequently in children of any skin type and in adults who have thick subcutaneous tissue.

Skin loss

At the other extreme, partial or complete loss of the skin graft can occur, most often in the first few months after surgery. Possible causes of graft loss include hematoma; seroma; infection; excessive graft pressure; and improper preparation of the recipient site, namely, removal of the periosteum under the skin graft. Skin graft losses may also be associated with other complicating medical factors that impair wound healing, such as smoking, diabetes mellitus, hyperglycemia, and local irradiation [24–27]. These factors are important to consider when counseling patients for primary BAHA surgery.

Revision BAHA surgery

Failure of osseointegration

The most common causes of fixture loss are, in order, trauma, incomplete fixture insertion, infection, and idiopathic. Fixture loss happens more commonly in children than adults because of the greater chance of trauma and incomplete fixture insertion in the pediatric population (Table 1). Trauma can dislodge the fixture or damage its connection to the abutment severely enough to require replacement.

The cause of fixture loss determines whether revision surgery is warranted. Traumatic cases are nearly always amenable to revision. Fixture loss from incomplete fixture insertion may be amenable to revision if there has been an increase in bone thickness. If infection was the cause of fixture loss, the infection must be resolved completely before considering replacement of the fixture. For severe infections, a CT of the temporal bone should

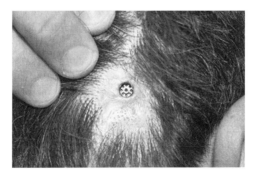

Fig. 3. Near total skin overgrowth of the abutment.

Table 1
Fixture loss rates from a selection of cohorts

Author	Number of fixtures	Early failure[a]	Late failure[b]	Trauma
Proops 1996 [10][c]	188	5 (3%)	12	2
Papsin et al 1997 [9][c]	32	3 (9%)	0	2
Reyes et al 2000 [3][d]	149	9 (6%)		4
Portmann et al 2001 [32]	87	3 (3%)	0	3
Wade 2002 [33][d]	76	2 (3%)		1
Zeitoun et al 2002 [7][c]	31 ears, but 56 fixtures implanted	5 (9%)	3	3
Priwin 2005 [34]	41	1 (%)	3	0

[a] Lack of osseointegration after the first stage of a two-stage procedure, or failure within the first year with a one-stage procedure.

[b] Failure 1 year after the first stage of a two-stage procedure, or 1 year after a one-stage procedure.

[c] Pediatric alone.

[d] Data not separated into early or late failures.

be performed after infection resolution to help determine the integrity of the underlying bone.

If a banked or sleeper fixture was used at the initial surgery, it can be used in cases of fixture loss of the primary implant. If the banked fixture failed to osseointegrate, then the likelihood of osseointegration failure is high with revision surgery.

When revision surgery is planned for a new fixture placement, an area of sufficient bone volume must be identified. The best chance for success is often found several millimeters posterior to the site of the original fixture. Once viable bone of sufficient volume is found, fixture placement proceeds as in the primary case. If necessary, surrounding soft tissue must be removed, as in the original procedure.

Bone overgrowth

Bony overgrowth, an uncommon cause of implant loss, is a complication that occurs exclusively in children. Bone can grow completely over the fixture or the abutment. Bone growth is sometimes advantageous if incomplete insertion is necessary, but more often than not, the bone needs to be removed because it interferes with device function.

Bone removal can be done with a curette or low-speed drill, using local or general anesthetic [20]. Care must be taken, however, not to damage or dislodge the fixture.

Skin reaction

A Grade 3 skin reaction [13] is defined as redness and moisture of the skin surrounding the abutment, with significant granulation tissue. Grade 3 reactions may, at times, be treated with conservative measures, such as oral and topical antibiotics, with local cauterization of the granulation tissue. If conservative measures fail, then it is recommended that the skin surrounding the abutment be removed and a skin graft applied, as outlined below.

Grade 4 reactions should be treated by removing both the skin surrounding the abutment, and the abutment with the fixture. A skin graft should be applied and a new implant may be placed in 3 months, if the area heals properly (Anders Tjellstrom, personal communication, 2006).

Skin overgrowth

Progressive development of excess subcutaneous tissue at the abutment site is the most common reason for revision BAHA surgery, especially in children. Skin overgrowth can occur at any time after the initial surgery. In one study [8], the investigators revised the skin flap every 3.5 years in patients aged 6 to 12 years because of skin overgrowth. No child below the age of 6 years required revision because of skin overgrowth.

The early stages of excessive skin growth may be arrested with the use of topical steroid cream (eg, Triamcinolone topical 0.5%) applied twice daily for 7 to 10 days. Local injection of steroid, in conjunction with topical application, should be considered in more severe cases. Steroid injection should not be used in any patient with known or suspected reason for delayed wound healing. Application of the steroid cream once a day should continue for several weeks, if there has been a favorable reaction to the initial steroid application.

Skin overgrowth may also be treated with in-office incision and removal of excessive tissue immediately surrounding the abutment. The edges of the incision may be cauterized with silver nitrate for hemostasis and to help prevent tissue regrowth.

When these conservative measures fail, the patient should be brought to the operating room for more extensive revision of the skin flap. Surgical revision of the skin flap involves removal of all tissue, including skin, down to the level of the periosteum. The authors advise against removal of only a superficial layer of excess subcutaneous tissue. Less than complete excision of all tissue to the level of the periosteum increases considerably the chance of redevelopment of skin overgrowth. The authors recommend removal of subcutaneous tissue in an area measuring at least 3.0 cm by 3.0 cm, centered on the abutment, rather than the 2.5 cm by 2.5 cm recommended at the time of the original surgery. The authors have found that skin overgrowth can recur in the 2.5 cm by 2.5 cm configuration, but rarely in the larger 3.0 cm by 3.0 cm configuration. As in the original procedure, the subcutaneous tissue should be widely undermined at the edge of the surrounding skin. After undermining the soft tissue, the skin is reapproximated to the periosteum using absorbable sutures.

A split thickness skin graft (STSG) is necessary to cover the area of removed tissue. Skin must be obtained from a separate donor site because all skin over the BAHA site is removed. Two popular donor sites include the volar aspect of the upper arm (ie, Thiersch graft) [28] and the lateral, upper thigh. The skin graft should be thin enough to remove any hair follicles. The skin graft is secured to the margins of the recipient site using interrupted absorbable sutures, and should be secured to the periosteum using absorbable sutures in a circumferential fashion around the base of the abutment.

Another option for treating skin overgrowth is the placement of a longer abutment. The standard abutment length is 5.5 mm. Cochlear Americas supplies a longer abutment (8.5 mm) that can be used in cases of chronic skin overgrowth. The abutment is removed and replaced by using the Countertorque Abutment Wrench and the UniGrip screwdriver (both instruments made by Bone Anchored Solutions, a Cochlear Group company). The abutment change can be performed in the office when there is partial or near-complete skin overgrowth (Fig. 3) of the abutment. When there is complete skin overgrowth, the patient should be brought to the operating room to remove some of the surrounding soft tissue.

Skin loss

Skin loss can occur with or without bone exposure. If underlying bone is not exposed, healing is delayed, but healing will often occur by secondary intention. Revision surgery is rarely needed in these cases.

Partial or complete loss of the skin graft with exposure of bone may require revision surgery. Fortunately, bone exposure is an uncommon occurrence. Loss of the skin flap can happen at any time, but occurs most commonly in the first 6 months after the creation of the flap. Conservative measures can be tried intitially for immunocompetent patients. All immunocompromised patients with bone exposure should undergo skin grafting. Conservative treatment consists of cleansing the bone and surrounding tissue daily with dilute vinegar solution followed by application of an antibacterial ointment. Skin grafting as outlined below should be considered if conservative measures fail after 2-3 weeks of treatment.

Small areas of bone exposure (eg, ≤ 1 cm^2) may, at times, be treated with skin grafting in the office. The best chance for success for covering these small defects is when granulation tissue surrounds the area of bone exposure. A full-thickness skin graft can be shaved with a number-10–scalpel blade from a hairless region in the postauricular area. The skin graft must be large enough to contact the surrounding granulation tissue. Before placement of the graft, the granulation tissue should be manipulated with a blunt instrument to cause local bleeding. A small amount of bleeding will facilitate graft "take." The graft is placed directly on bone and granulation tissue, without the need for suturing. It is bolstered with gauze and a healing cap for 7 days. After removal of the bolster, antibiotic ointment is applied gently to the area twice daily for 7 days. If in-office skin grafting fails, the area of bone exposure must be treated with local flaps or skin grafting in the operating room.

Large or complete loss of the skin graft with bone exposure requires salvage with a local flap. Coverage of bone is important to prevent osteomyelitis. In addition, loss of the graft can delay use of the device for several months [29]. Several options are available to cover bone and create a viable skin–implant interface. For smaller defects, local skin advancement flaps are an option. The advancement flap is created by making two parallel incisions extending out from the area of bone exposure. The width of the flap should be slightly wider than the area of bone exposure. As with any advancement flap, thorough undermining is necessary to ensure a tension-free graft. The distal end of the flap should be thinned and depilated to create a hairless area of skin.

The largest defects require creation of local rotation flaps with a STSG. One option is a galeal rotation flap [29]. The galeal flap is supplied by the occipital artery [30] and is created by making a linear incision extended posteriorly into the scalp from the defect. The scalp is separated from the pericranium and the galea is then dissected sharply in a subfollicular plane. A posteriorly based galeal flap is designed and then rotated over the exposed bone. The galeal flap is thin, and should be covered with a STSG from either the upper arm or lateral thigh.

The superficial temporal parietal fascia (STPF) flap is another reliable flap that can be used to cover areas of exposed bone after BAHA surgery. STPF lies superficial to the deep temporal fascia covering the temporalis muscle, and continues as the galea beyond the limits of the temporal fossa. The STPF flap is supplied by the superficial temporal artery and vein, with the flap hinged in the region of the zygomatic arch. To create the flap, a vertical skin incision is made, starting at the zygomatic arch a few centimeters anterior to the root of the auricle. The incision is carried as far superiorly as necessary to obtain a graft of sufficient length. As with the galeal flap, the STPF flap is thin and should be covered with an STSG [31].

Summary

Although BAHA surgery is not difficult, the surgeon must observe meticulous technique to prevent complications. The success rate of BAHA fixture osseointegration has improved since the technique for BAHA insertion was developed in 1977. The most common reasons for failure of osseointegration after either a primary or a revision procedure include trauma, incomplete insertion, and infection. Skin overgrowth continues to be a problem in both children and adults, and is the most common reason for revision BAHA surgery.

References

[1] Battista RA, Ho SY. The bone-anchored hearing device (BAHA). Operative techniques. Otolarygol Head Neck Surg 2003;14(4):272–6.

[2] Tjellström A, Granstrom G. One-stage procedure to establish osseointegration: a zero to five years follow-up report. J Laryngol Otol 1995;109(7):593–8.

[3] Reyes RA, Tjellström A, Granstrom G. Evaluation of implant losses and skin reactions around extraoral bone-anchored implants: A 0- to 8-year follow-up. Otolaryngol Head Neck Surg 2000;122(2):272–6.

[4] Tjellström A, Granstrom G. Long-term follow-up with the bone-anchored hearing aid: a review of the first 100 patients between 1977 and 1985. Ear Nose Throat J 1994;73(2):112–4.

[5] Jacobsson M, Albrektsson T, Tjellström A. Tissue-integrated implants in children. Int J Pediatr Otorhinolaryngol 1992;24(3):235–43.

[6] Portmann D, Boudard P, Herman D. Anatomical results with titanium implants in the mastoid region. Ear Nose Throat J 1997;76(4):231–4, 6.

[7] Zeitoun H, De R, Thompson SD, et al. Osseointegrated implants in the management of childhood ear abnormalities: with particular emphasis on complications. J Laryngol Otol 2002;116(2):87–91.

[8] Granstrom G, Bergstrom K, Odersjo M, et al. Osseointegrated implants in children: experience from our first 100 patients. Otolaryngol Head Neck Surg 2001;125(1):85–92.

[9] Papsin BC, Sirimanna TK, Albert DM, et al. Surgical experience with bone-anchored hearing aids in children. Laryngoscope 1997;107(6):801–6.

[10] Proops DW. The Birmingham bone anchored hearing aid programme: surgical methods and complications. J Laryngol Otol Suppl 1996;21:7–12.

[11] Granstrom G, Tjellström A. Effects of irradiation on osseointegration before and after implant placement: a report of three cases. Int J Oral Maxillofac Implants 1997;12(4):547–51.

[12] Granstrom G, Tjellström A, Branemark PI. Osseointegrated implants in irradiated bone: a case-controlled study using adjunctive hyperbaric oxygen therapy. J Oral Maxillofac Surg 1999;57(5):493–9.

[13] Holgers KM, Tjellström A, Bjursten LM, et al. Soft tissue reactions around percutaneous implants: a clinical study on skin-penetrating titanium implants used for bone-anchored auricular prostheses. Int J Oral Maxillofac Implants 1987;2(1):35–9.

[14] Tjellström A, Hakansson B. The bone-anchored hearing aid. Design principles, indications, and long-term clinical results. Otolaryngol Clin North Am 1995;28(1):53–72.

[15] Holgers KM, Tjellström A, Bjursten LM, et al. Soft tissue reactions around percutaneous implants: a clinical study of soft tissue conditions around skin-penetrating titanium implants for bone-anchored hearing aids. Am J Otol 1988;9(1):56–9.

[16] Granstrom G, Tjellström A. The bone-anchored hearing aid (BAHA) in children with auricular malformations. Ear Nose Throat J 1997;76(4):238–40, 42, 44–7.

[17] Bejar-Solar I, Rosete M, de Jesus Madrazo M, et al. Percutaneous bone-anchored hearing aids at a pediatric institution. Otolaryngol Head Neck Surg 2000;122(6):887–91.

[18] Stevenson DS, Proops DW, Wake MJ, et al. Osseointegrated implants in the management of childhood ear abnormalities: the initial Birmingham experience. J Laryngol Otol 1993; 107(6):502–9.

[19] Wazen JJ, Caruso M, Tjellström A. Long-term results with the titanium bone-anchored hearing aid: the US experience. Am J Otol 1998;19(6):737–41.

[20] Sunkaraneni VS, Gray RF. Bony overgrowth onto fixture component of a bone-anchored hearing aid. J Laryngol Otol 2004;118(8):643–4.

[21] Holgers KM, Roupe G, Tjellström A, et al. Clinical, immunological and bacteriological evaluation of adverse reactions to skin-penetrating titanium implants in the head and neck region. Contact Dermatitis 1992;27(1):1–7.

[22] Scholz M, Eufinger H, Anders A, et al. Intracerebral abscess after abutment change of a bone anchored hearing aid (BAHA). Otol Neurotol 2003;24(6):896–9.

[23] Deitmer T, Krassort M, Hartmann S. [Two rare complications in patients with bone-anchored hearing aids]. Laryngorhinootologie 2003;82(3):162–5.

[24] Krueger JK, Rohrich RJ. Clearing the smoke: the scientific rationale for tobacco abstention with plastic surgery. Plast Reconstr Surg 2001;108(4):1063–73 [discussion: 74–7].

[25] Burns JL, Mancoll JS, Phillips LG. Impairments to wound healing. Clin Plast Surg 2003; 30(1):47–56.

[26] Hoogwerf BJ. Postoperative management of the diabetic patient. Med Clin North Am 2001; 85(5):1213–28.

[27] Mowlavi A, Andrews K, Milner S, et al. The effects of hyperglycemia on skin graft survival in the burn patient. Ann Plast Surg 2000;45(6):629–32.

[28] Harvey SA. Skin grafting in otology. Laryngoscope 1997;107(9):1199–202.

[29] Snyder MC, Moore GF, Johnson PJ. The use of full-thickness skin grafts for the skin-abutment interface around bone-anchored hearing aids. Otol Neurotol 2003;24(2):255–8.

[30] de Magalhaes RP, Brandao LG, Magalhaes MG, et al. Galeal pedicle flap of the occipital region for pharynx reconstruction: anatomic and clinical considerations. Plast Reconstr Surg 1998;102(6):2124–8.

[31] Mathes SJ, Nahai F. Reconstructive surgery: principles, anatomy and technique. New York: Churchill Livingstone, Inc.; 1997.

[32] Portmann D, Boudard P, Vdovytsya O. [Bone-anchored hearing aids BAHA: 10 years' experience]. Rev Stomatol Chir Maxillofac 2001;102(5):274–7.

[33] Wade PS, Halik JJ, Werger JP, et al. Ten-year experience with percutaneous bone-anchored hearing aids: a 3- to 10-year follow-up Markham Stouffville Hospital, 1990 to 2000. J Otolaryngol 2002;31(2):80–4.

[34] Priwin C, Granstrom G. The bone-anchored hearing aid in children: a surgical and question-naire follow-up study. Otolaryngol Head Neck Surg 2005;132(4):559–65.

ELSEVIER
SAUNDERS

Otolaryngol Clin N Am
39 (2006) 815–832

OTOLARYNGOLOGIC
CLINICS
OF NORTH AMERICA

Revision Facial Nerve Surgery

Arvind Kumar, MD[a,b,c,d,*], John Ryzenman, MD[c],
Arlene Barr, MD[e]

[a]Department of Otolaryngology–Head and Neck Surgery, University of Illinois,
Chicago, IL, USA
[b]Department of Neurosurgery, University of Illinois, Chicago, IL, USA
[c]Department of Otolaryngology Head and Neck Surgery, Northwestern University Feinberg
School of Medicine, 303 East Chicago Avenue, Searle 12-561, Chicago, IL 60611, USA
[d]Ear Institute of Chicago, LLC, Hinsdale, IL, USA
[e]Department of Neurology and Rehabilitation, University of Illinois at Chicago,
Chicago, IL, USA

Transection of the facial nerve can result from blunt or penetrating trauma to the face or temporal bone. It can also occur accidentally during surgery, or as a planned surgical procedure carried out in the interest of eradicating disease. If transection is recognized at surgery, direct anastomosis or cable grafting is the procedure of choice. Immediate nerve repair offers the best chance for recovery, which usually begins within 9 to 12 months [1]. What if at the end of this period there is neither clinical nor electrical evidence of recovery? A report by May and colleagues [2] discussed the investigation and management of such a case; however, this specific problem has not been reviewed in the English language since then. This article presents two similar cases with poor outcomes. The authors review current understanding of the immediate and long-term changes that occur in the neuron, axon, and muscle after injury to the nerve, and the underlying pathology that led to graft failure. They also evaluate the applicable surgical options described in the literature and the diagnostic test results that help in selecting the most appropriate surgical procedure in these cases.

* Corresponding author.
Department of Otolaryngology Head and Neck Surgery, Northwestern University Feinberg
School of Medicine, 303 East Chicago Avenue, Searle 12-561, Chicago, IL 60611, USA.

0030-6665/06/$ - see front matter © 2006 Elsevier Inc. All rights reserved.
doi:10.1016/j.otc.2006.04.002   *oto.theclinics.com*

Materials and methods

Patient # 1

A 20-year-old man sustained a blow to the left side of his head, and, as a result, he lost consciousness for several hours. In the emergency room he was noted to have a left infranuclear facial paralysis and bleeding from the ipsilateral ear. The patient was confined to the intensive care unit for an extended period because of other serious body injuries. He sought consultation for his left facial paralysis and hearing loss 2 months after the original injury. Physical examination of the head and neck showed no abnormality, except for a complete left infranuclear facial paralysis. The Rinne was negative on the left and the Weber lateralized to the left. An audiometric evaluation confirmed a conductive hearing loss on the left side. A CT scan of the temporal bone showed an otic capsule sparing longitudinal fracture of the left temporal bone. In an effort to understand the nature of the lesion causing the paralysis, in the face of a CT-scan–confirmed intact fallopian canal, MRI with contrast of the brain and facial nerve were obtained. The MRI was read by the neuroradiologist as showing an intraneural hematoma at the geniculate ganglion. The facial nerve was decompressed by way of a transmastoid-subtemporal approach. The incus was found to be dislocated and was therefore removed. To access the geniculate ganglion, the head of the malleus was amputated. Examination of the fallopian canal from the meatal foramen to the second genu failed to show spicules or a fracture line traversing the canal. The fallopian canal was opened from just distal to the meatal foramen to the second genu, and, in view of the findings noted on the MRI scan, this segment of the nerve was excised. A great auricular nerve graft was approximated to the two ends of the transected facial nerve. No sutures were used to stabilize the anastomoses, and no glues were used at the anastomotic sites. A malleus-stapes assembly was placed through the facial recess and the incision closed. Two months later, an audiogram showed closure of the air-bone gap to within 15 dB of bone scores. Histologic examination of the nerve specimen showed dense fibrosis in the geniculate ganglion.

When the patient returned 6 months later, there was no clinical or electrophysiologic evidence of recovery. His cornea was reported normal by the ophthalmologist, and with eye closure a good Bell's phenomenon was noted. The patient returned for a follow-up examination 3 years later and an evaluation of facial nerve function showed a complete paralysis on the left side. He did not wish to undergo any electromyography (EMG) studies on this visit; nor did he agree to any further surgery.

Patient # 2

Over the course of 4 years, an 18-year-old woman developed a progressive right-sided facial paralysis. She did not admit to any loss of hearing in the right ear, or to any loss of taste, or tearing. During the course of a pregnancy

6 months earlier, she had noted a more rapid progression of the facial paralysis. Examination of the head and neck showed a complete right infranuclear facial paralysis but no other abnormalities. Tuning fork tests showed positive Rinne on both sides and the Weber lateralized to the right. A CT scan of the temporal bone (Fig. 1A,C) and an MRI brain scan (Fig. 1B,D) confirmed a tumor in the region of the geniculate ganglion, thought to be a facial nerve schwannoma. An EMG showed fibrillation potentials in all areas of the face. In May 2002, the tumor was resected via a right transmastoid-subtemporal approach with primary cable grafting using the great auricular nerve. No sutures were used to anchor the graft. The extent of the tumor mass was judged visually, rather than with frozen

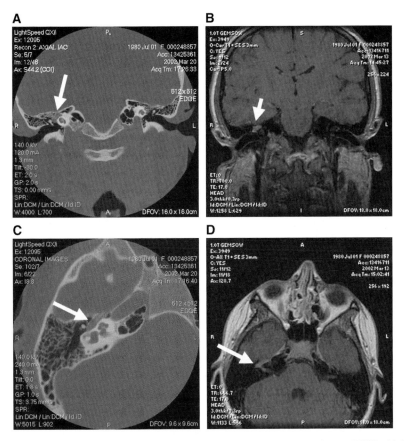

Fig. 1. (*A*) and (*B*) Preoperative coronal CT and MRI for patient #2. MRI image, T1WI with IV contrast demonstrates enlargement and homogeneous contrast enhancement of the geniculate ganglion of the right facial nerve (*small arrow*). Coronal noncontrast CT demonstrates a soft tissue mass expanding the bone surrounding the geniculate ganglion of the right facial nerve (*large arrow*). (*C*) and (*D*) Preoperative axial CT and MRI for patient #2 demonstrate enlargement of the region of the geniculate ganglion and tympanic segment of the right facial nerve canal (*arrows*).

section. The ossicular reconstruction was completed using a Total Ossicular Replacement Prosthesis (TORP). Her postoperative recovery was unremarkable, and an audiogram done 3 months later showed a 10 dB conductive hearing loss. The pathology report confirmed a diagnosis of "meningothelial and psammomatous meningioma." This diagnosis was reached by two independent pathologists at two different institutions.

Three years later she still has a complete right infranuclear facial paralysis. In addition, there is blephroptosis on the right side, a wider palpebral fissure on the right, inadequate closure of the right eye, collapse of the nasal ala on the right, and inadequacy of the oral sphincter upon puffing the cheeks (Fig. 2). These observations correspond with the patient's complaints of drooling liquids from the angle of the mouth, and excessive tearing. An ophthalmologic consultation reported no corneal ulcers and a good Bell's

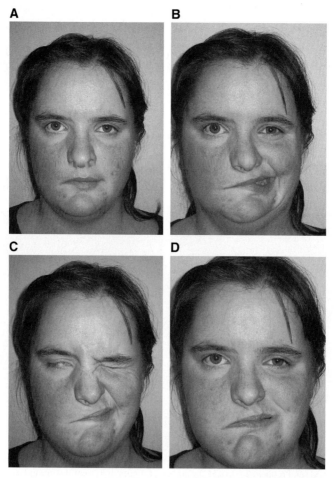

Fig. 2. Facial function 3 years postoperatively for patient #2.

phenomenon. An EMG study showed no motor unit action potentials, and "clear insertional activity, fibrillations and positive sharp waves." An MRI scan showed a recurrent tumor in the right labyrinthine segment of the nerve (Fig. 3). A CT scan of the right temporal bone showed postsurgical changes and a "mild to moderate enlargement of the right facial canal, particularly in the labyrinthine segment with a focus of increased density... most likely hyperostotic changes compatible with the known recurrent perigenicular meningioma."

Discussion

Acute changes in neuron, axon, and muscle after nerve injury

An understanding of the postinjury changes that occur in the facial nerve neuron, its axon, and the muscles innervated by it is important for understanding the rationale for the current rehabilitative algorithms. Within 1 to 2 days of injury to the nerve, its cell body swells, its nucleus moves peripherally, and there is loss of Nissl substance (chromatolysis); this activity reaches its peak in about 2 weeks (Fig. 4). Electron microscopic studies have shown that the number of cellular organelles also increased [3]. These neuronal changes are accompanied by changes in the microenvironment of the facial nucleus. Within 24 hours, microglia, which are phagocytic cells of the central nervous system, are stimulated, move into direct contact with injured neurons, and displace synaptic input. This phenomenon is known as *synaptic stripping* [3]. Astrocytes, which provide physical and metabolic support to cells of the central nervous system, show rapid induction of growth

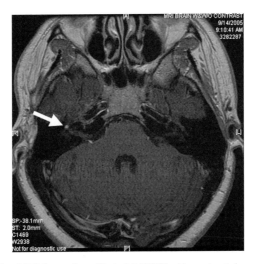

Fig. 3. Postoperative MRI for patient #2. Axial T1WI with contrast demonstrates punctuate contrast enhancement in the right geniculate ganglion, indicating residual meningioma (*arrow*).

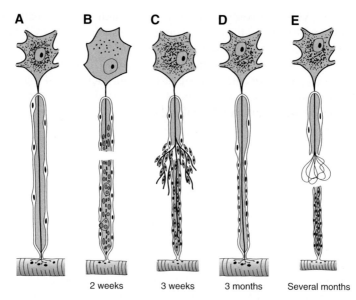

Fig. 4. Main changes that take place in an injured nerve fiber. (*A*) Normal nerve fiber, with its perikaryon and the effector cell (striated skeletal muscle). Note the position of the neuron nucleus and the number and distribution of Nissl bodies. (*B*) When the fiber is injured, the neuronal nucleus moves to the cell periphery, and the number of Nissl bodies is greatly reduced. The nerve fiber distal to the injury degenerates along with its myelin sheath. Debris is phagocytosed by macrophages. (*C*) The muscle fiber shows pronounced disuse atrophy. Schwann cells proliferate, forming a compact cord penetrated by the growing axon. The axon grows at a rate of 3mm/day. (*D*) In this example, the nerve fiber regeneration was successful. Note that the muscle fiber was also regenerated after receiving nerve stimuli. (*E*) When the axons do not penetrate the cord of Schwann cells, its growth is disorganized. (*Adapted from* Ross MH, Romrell LJ, Kaye GI. Response of neurons to injury. In: Ross MH, Romrell LJ, Kaye GI, editors. Histology: a text and atlas. Ross's 3rd edition. Baltimore, Maryland: Williams and Wilkins; 1995. p. 284.)

factors and gradually replace microglia on the neuronal surface. With successful nerve regeneration, the astrocytes retract and the neuronal surface is repopulated with synaptic terminals [3].

Although there is no measurable proliferation of capillaries, a functional activation of local vasculature occurs, so that regenerating motor neurons receive additional energy and building materials. These changes are thought to facilitate the production of new axoplasm, and, teleologically, this is sound and acceptable. However, the experimental observations of Stennert [4] provide a central cause for postrecovery synkinesis. In a cohort of 12 young female rats, six underwent a facio-facial anastomosis and the other six served as a control group. Twenty-seven months later, all animals underwent surgical exposure of the peripheral facial nerve branches for application of different colored retrograde tracers: Di I (red), FG (white), and FB (blue). One week later, all rats were perfused, their brains removed, and the brainstem sections examined under a fluorescent microscope, using different UV filters. The unoperated rats showed normal somatotopic organization of the corresponding motor neurons inside the facial nucleus as red, white, and blue coherent clusters (Fig. 5). The operated rats showed loss of the clusterlike somatotopic organization and several motor neurons showed a mixture of tracer colors (Fig. 6).

During regeneration, there is an overall increase in transport of protein in the axon, and the increased flow of axoplasm leads to a considerable enlargement of the axon tip of the proximal nerve segment. An accumulation of signaling molecules at the distal end of the proximal segment is also evident; this is known as the *growth cone*. Within a week of injury, bundles of axonal sprouts (filopodia) grow into the distal segment of the transected nerve. This neurite outgrowth can be inhibited by several factors, including the persistence of myelin in the distal segment [3].

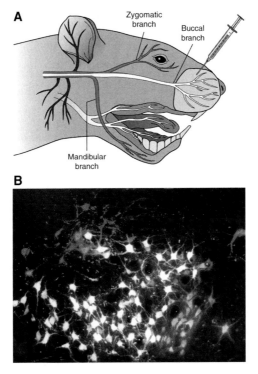

Fig. 5. (*A*) Injection of different retrograde tracers into the facial muscles. (*Adapted from* Stennert E. Synkineses and the autoparalytic syndrome. In: The facial palsies–complementary approaches. 1st edition. Utrecht, The Netherlands: Lemma Publishers; 2005. p. 117–133; with permission.) (*B*) Normal somatotopic clusterlike organization of the facial nucleus after retrograde tracing in nonoperated control. (*Adapted from* Dohm S, Streppel M, Guntinas-Lichius O, et al. Local application of extracellular matrix proteins fails to reduce the number of axonal branches after varying reconstructive surgery on rat facial nerve. Restor Neurol Neurosci 2000;16:117–26; with permission.)

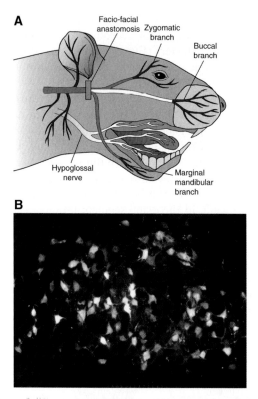

Fig. 6. (*A*) Injection of different retrograde tracers into the facial muscles after facio-facial anastomosis. (*Adapted from* Stennert E. Synkineses and the autoparalytic syndrome. In: The facial palsies–complementary approaches. 1st edition. Utrecht, The Netherlands: Lemma Publishers; 2005. p. 117–133; with permission.) (*B*) Facial nucleus 8 weeks after facio-facial anastomosis and 10 days after identical triple retrograde labeling as in Fig. 5 (*B*). Note the complete loss of somatotopic organization of the facial nucleus; motor neurons are scattered throughout the whole nucleus. (*Adapted from* Dohm, S, Streppel M, Guntinas-Lichius O, et al. Local application of extracellular matrix proteins fails to reduce the number of axonal branches after varying reconstructive surgery on rat facial nerve. Restor Neurol Neurosci 2000;16:117–26; with permission.)

Nerve fibers disconnected from their neuron begin to degenerate within hours of the injury. However, nerve conductivity and axonal transport in the distal segment are preserved for several days, and this is the basis for electrical tests such as electroneurography. Within the first 2 to 3 days, there is axolysis and proliferation of Schwann cells (wallerian degeneration). The myelin sheath also fragments and there is a breakdown of the blood-nerve barrier. Thus, circulating monocytes enter the nerve parenchyma, transform into tissue macrophages, and, together with Schwann cells, phagocytose axonal and myelin fragments. Proliferating Schwann cells form tubular structures within the endoneurial tubes (Bands of Büngner) and these strongly support axonal regeneration. The breakdown of the blood-brain barrier

allows serum growth factors, such as transferrin, to enter the nerve parenchyma and facilitate axonal regeneration (Fig. 7).

The morphologic change at the myoneural junction is that the primary
synaptic cleft becomes shallower and the secondary synaptic clefts become
shallower and wider (Fig. 8). The basal lamina of the target muscle persists;
this structure is known to be a vital factor in the formation of new synaptic
connections during reinnervation.

A number of morphologic changes also occur in a denervated muscle.
The one most widely recognized, both in terms of number and types of

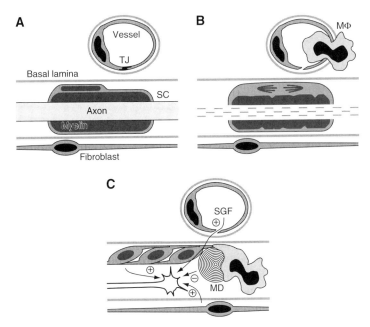

Fig. 7. Cellular changes in the injured and regenerating peripheral nerve. (*A*) Longitudinal section through a normal neural tube with myelinated motor axons and associated Schwann cells
(SC) surrounded by basal lamina. The tight junctions (TJ) of the adjacent endoneurial vessels
form the structural basis of the blood-nerve barrier in the normal, uninjured peripheral nerve.
(*B*) Axonal injury causes a rapid degeneration of the distal, disconnected axon, followed by a de-
stabilization of the associated myelin and Schwann cell proliferation. Axonal degeneration also
leads to a breakdown of the blood-nerve barrier and adhesion of circulating monocytes, which
transform into tissue macrophages (MO) and later invade the endoneurial tubes. (*C*) Proliferating Schwann cells form endoneurial Büngner bands that strongly support axonal regeneration. They are assisted by adjacent fibroblasts that provide neurotrophic factors and
nutritional material for axonal growth. The absence of the blood-nerve barrier also provides
access for serum growth factors (SGF), such as transferrin, to aid ongoing axonal regeneration.
In contrast, the myelin debris (MD) contains a number of inhibitory molecules that block neurite outgrowth. The removal of myelin by macrophages plays a central role in promoting nerve
regeneration. (*Adapted from* May M, Gantz B, Hughes G. Management of failed nerve graft
following facial nerve resection for facial nerve neurofibroma. Head Neck Surg 1987;9:184–7;
with permission.)

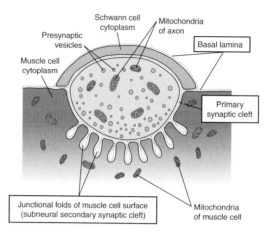

Fig. 8. The neuromuscular junction. An axon is shown making contact with the muscle cell. Note how the junctional folds of the muscle cell augment the surface area within the synaptic cleft. The basal lamina extends throughout the cleft area. The cytoplasm of the Schwann cell is shown covering the axon terminal. (*Adapted from* Ross MH, Romrell LJ, Kaye GI. Response of neurons to injury. In: Ross MH, Romrell LJ, Kaye GI, editors. Histology: a text and atlas. Ross's. 3rd edition. Baltimore, Maryland: Williams and Wilkins; 1995. p. 284.)

fibers, is pronounced muscle atrophy. Muscle atrophy of 20% to 90% of baseline has been reported [5]. Histologically, there is a well-documented increase in the number of satellite cells (Fig. 9) [6]. These satellite cells are myogenic precursors and could be involved in the restoration of muscle mass after reinnervation. Acetylcholine receptors are spread over the surface of the denervated muscle. Ultimately, many denervated muscle fibers are replaced by fat cells and connective tissue. Neuromuscular changes following nerve transection are summarized in Table 1. All this information is, for the most part, derived from observations made on limb musculature in small animals, and, in fact, very little research has been done on muscles innervated by the facial nerve [6].

Chronic changes in the facial nerve, nucleus, and muscle after long-term injury

Because the problem the authors are confronted with is the management of long-term facial paralysis, it is pertinent to discuss the effects of long-term denervation on the neuron, proximal segment, distal segment, myoneural junction, and muscle. Information on this is sparse in the literature, particularly with reference to the facial nerve. The experimental work of Stennert [4] provides an understanding of changes that occur at the nuclear level of a transected nerve, as described earlier.

Limited knowledge exists of the long-term effects of nerve transection on the proximal segment of the injured nerve. The hitherto unknown effects of stretch injury on the proximal segment in humans have been described by

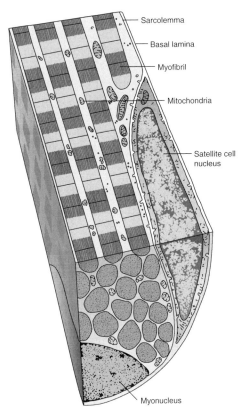

Fig. 9. A muscle-fiber–satellite-cell complex. Note that the satellite cell and the muscle fiber are enclosed within a common basal lamina. (*Adapted from* Carlson BM. Skeletal muscle-denervation, reinnervation, and muscle transplantation. In: The facial nerve. May's 2nd edition. New York: Thieme; 2000. p. 81–94.)

Felix and colleagues [7]. They noted that the proximal segment showed dense retrograde fibrosis for varying distances along the length of the nerve.

Ylikoski and colleagues [8] have described long-term changes in the distal segment of the human facial nerve. They studied the distal segment of five human facial nerves that had been transected 17 days earlier in one subject, 3 months earlier in two subjects, 7 months earlier in one subject, and 30 months earlier in one subject.

All the pathologic specimens were studied by light and electron microscopy. All five subjects underwent XII-VII anastomosis. The histopathologic findings, follow-up periods, and results of the anastomosis are summarized in Table 2. The most striking findings were seen in subject # 4, in whom the result was poor and the distal segment showed total fibrosis, even though the nerve anastomosis was done just 7 months after transection. This result contrasts with subject # 5, in whom there was only slight endoneurial fibrosis 30 months after transection, and whose functional result was "much

Table 1
Summary of the changes that occur in the neuromuscular complex

Structure	Pathologic changes	Time course
Cell body	Cell body swells and nucleus marginalizes. There is chromatolysis, hyperplasia of cellular organelles, and loss of somatotopic organization.	1 to 2 days
Microglia	Microglia contact affected neurons and cause synaptic stripping. They are replaced by astrocytes that promote growth factors and metabolic support.	Within 24 hours
Proximal axon	Axoplasm increases and proximal tip engorges (growth cone). Filopodia sprout and seek out endoneurial tubules.	Hours to days
Distal axon	Axonal transport is preserved for 48–72 hours. Axolysis and Scwhann cells proliferate, myelin sheaths fragment and are phagocytosed by microglia. Bands of Büngner form.	Days
Myoneural junction	Primary and secondary synaptic clefts become shallow. Basal lamina is scaffold for muscle regeneration and reorganization of myoneural junctions.	Days to weeks
Muscle	Muscle atrophy and hypoplasia ensue within months. Satellite cells multiply and differentiate to restore muscle mass. Acetylcholine receptors spread out then regroup to accept incoming regenerated nerve.	Weeks to months

improved" 6 months after anastomosis. It appears, therefore, that endoneurial fibrosis is not a function of time, but is certainly an impediment to regeneration, as shown by this study and the study by Felix and colleagues [7]. Nevertheless, Carlson [6] is of the opinion that "a significant factor that determines the level of success of reinnervation of a denervated muscle is the condition of the distal pathways through which the regenerating axons must pass." He drew particular attention to the state of the basal lamina at the myoneural junction (see Fig. 8). If this structure is filled with deposits of collagen, the outgrowth of regenerating axons is inhibited.

Data on long-term changes at the myoneural junction and in human facial muscles are scanty. As for the histopathology of denervated muscle, Belal [9] provided one of the first reports on the structure of human muscle in facial paralysis. He studied the postauricular and stapedius muscles of 14 subjects whose facial nerves had been injured. The paralysis occurred during the course of surgery (n = 8), or the subjects developed Bell's palsy (n = 3), or herpes zoster (n = 1), or tumors (n = 2), or malignant external otitis (n = 1). The duration of the paralysis ranged from 10 days to 6 years (Table 3). The pathologic changes were correlated neither to the underlying cause nor to any EMG studies that may have been done. Without such a correlation, these data, though valuable in themselves, do not help in the management decisions of long-term paralysis.

Bardosi [10] reported subsequently on the ultrastructure of normal and denervated human facial muscle. Facial muscle biopsies were obtained from 25 subjects ranging in age from 14 to 89 years. In this cohort, 17

Table 2
Summary of clinical and histopathologic data of five subjects who underwent hypoglossal-facial anastomosis

Case	Age	Sex	Diagnosis	Postop. time from facial nerve severance	Histopathologic findings in distal stump of facial nerve	Clinical results of re-innervation surgery	Follow-up time
1	32	F	Acoustic neuroma	17 days	Wallerian degeneration in progress, all stages present; sensory fibers intact	Slightly improved function	6 months
2	31	M	Meningioma	3 months	Major portion degenerated with scattered surviving fibers; increased endoneurial fibrosis; bands of Büngner; intact sensory bundle	Much improved function	18 months
3	47	F	Meningioma	3 months	Degeneration of all nerve fibers; increased endoneurial fibrosis; bands of Büngner	Much improved function	4 years
4	28	F	Meningioma	7 months	Total fibrotic change	No improvement	3 years
5	32	F	Middle ear cholesteatoma with intracranial extension	30 months	Nerve trunk of multifascicular type; degeneration of myelinated fibers except a few (vagus branch); slight endoneurial fibrosis; bands of Büngner	Much improved function	6 months

Data from Ylikoski J, Hitselberger WE, House WF, et al. Degenerative changes in the distal stump of the severed human facial nerve. Acta Otolaryngol 1981; 92:239–248.

Table 3
Natural history of denervation atrophy

Time course	Pathologic changes
10 days	Chains of subsarcolemmal nuclei
	Infoldings of nucleolar membrane
	No myofibrillar changes
17 days	Focal myofibrillar disruption
	Fragmentation of Z-line
	Subsarcolemmal mitochondrial hyperplasia
	Indentations of sarcolemma
6 weeks	Small-group atrophy of myofibrils
	Central migration of nuclei
	Disruption of some myofibrils
13 months	Large-group atrophy of myofibrils
	Degenerated myofibrils
	Increased collagen filaments
6 years	Large-group atrophy of myofibrils
	Dissociation of plasma and basement membranes
	Increased collagen filaments

Data from Kreutzberg GW, Raivich G. Neurobiology of regeneration and degeneration. In: The facial nerve. May's 2nd edition. New York: Thieme; 2000. p. 67–79.

subjects had undergone EMG tests and all showed evidence of denervation. The duration of facial paralysis in these 17 subjects ranged from 1 month to 36 years. However, no mention was made of the cause of the paralysis. The investigators found that the ultrastructure of normal human facial muscles did not differ in any respect from normal human striated muscle. The main difference between denervated and normal muscle was the presence of "a broad spectrum of inclusion bodies" in the former.

The success of reinnervation has been attributed for the most part to the condition of the muscle itself. Denervation muscle atrophy is well recognized clinically and histopathologically, and the principal cause is a reduction in the size and number of myofibrils within the muscle fiber [6]. Denervated muscles also undergo capillary reduction and connective tissue deposition (secondary atrophy); these changes could also add to the resistance to reinnervation [6].

Unfortunately, even with this background information, clinicians still have many questions:

- At what point after denervation does the facial musculature become incapable of reinnervation?
- Does the degree of muscle fiber atrophy influence its ability to reinnervate?
- Can regenerating fibers reach chronically denervated facial muscles?
- If regenerating nerve fibers can reach atrophic muscles, can functional neuromuscular junctions form?
- Can atrophic muscle fibers respond to the trophic influence of regenerating nerves?

The successful outcomes reported by Conley and colleagues [5] and Gagnon and Molina-Negro [11] in subjects with long-term paralysis suggest that although the above questions cannot be answered based on current clinical or experimental data, careful clinical observations can and should continue to be made, colleagues from radiology, neurology, and pathology should be closely involved, and patients should continue to be treated empirically. In most cases of long-term facial paralysis, it would be beneficial to know if a dynamic reinnervation is likely to succeed.

To this end, the authors would like to evaluate preoperatively the changes described above, in the neuron, the proximal nerve segment, the distal segment, the myoneural junction, and the denervated muscle. In practical terms, the only structure that can be studied preoperatively is the muscle, with EMG. On needle EMG, the first sign of axonal loss in the facial nerve is the development of abnormal spontaneous activity (ie, fibrillations and positive sharp waves that usually appear within 10 to 14 days of axonal transaction) [12]. Fibrillation potentials are short duration (1–5 milliseconds) biphasic or triphasic discharges of 20 to 500 μV amplitude. Positive sharp waves have an initial sharp positive deflection followed by a longer-lasting negative waveform; these can last up to 100 milliseconds and have amplitudes in the same range as fibrillation potentials. The fibrillation or positive sharp wave from each muscle fiber usually has a rhythmic discharge. However, the aggregate of fibrillations and positive sharp waves from multiple muscle fibers in the recording range of the needle electrode produce a sound over the amplifier that has been likened to that of "wrinkling tissue paper" [13]. Most investigators agree that fibrillations and positive sharp waves are a result of hyperexcitabilty in the denervated membrane of single muscle fibers [14]. Although the mechanisms underlying muscle and nerve membrane abnormalities after transection are not understood completely, there is increasing evidence that ion channel abnormalities are involved [15,16].

Fibrillations and positive sharp waves continue to be present in muscle on needle EMG until there is either reinnervation or atrophy with replacement by connective tissue [14]. Waveform size is not a universally accepted indicator of the amount of viable muscle or age of the lesion because of limitations associated with the distance of the recording needle electrode from the discharging muscle membrane, variation in fiber size, and sampling error. Measurement of the evoked compound muscle action potential amplitude on a nerve conduction study remains the standard method for assessing the amount of viable muscle. With progressive reinnervation (or progressive muscle atrophy), the number of positive sharp waves and fibrillation potentials decreases. Eventually, the size of the discharges diminishes; the decrease in size may be due to multiple factors, such as muscle atrophy or distance from the recording needle [17].

During reinnervation, reliable and predictable changes occur in the morphology of motor unit action potentials evoked from the reinnervated muscles. Larger, more complex motor unit action potential waveforms develop as a consequence of axonal sprouting and the increase in the number of muscle fibers receiving nerve supply from a single motor neuron. The number of functioning motor units in the recording territory of the needle EMG electrode depends on the degree of successful reinnervation. With more successful reinnervation, there are more functioning motor units. The term applied to the aggregate of motor units is "recruitment." Recruitment is reduced when the number of motor units is less than would be seen in a normal muscle.

The causes of failure of return of function in the two cases discussed appear clear in hindsight. In the first case, the seminal observations of Felix [7] showed that in stretch injuries of the facial nerve, such as occur in longitudinal or otic capsule sparing fractures, there is extensive endoneurial fibrosis proximal and distal to the geniculate ganglion. This fibrosis prevents the growth of axonal sprouts into the Bands of Büngner in the nerve segment distal to the intervening band of fibrosis. These findings were unavailable at the time of the first patient's surgery, and thus the nerve anastomosis was made proximally and distally to an area of the nerve that was fibrotic. Thus, failure of return of function was inevitable. Clearly, failure in the second case was due to the residual tumor at the proximal anastomotic site (see Fig. 3).

Management

Conley and May [18] classified facial restoration procedures into dynamic (Groups I-III) and static or adjunctive ones (Groups IV-VI). The details of individual procedures are summarized in Table 4. Most surgeons

Table 4
Classification of facial restoration procedures

Group	Type	Procedure
1	Dynamic	Facio-facial grafts: end-to-end, interposition, or double cable
2	Dynamic	Cranial nerve substitution: XII-VII, XII-VII jump, VII-VII (cross facial)
3	Dynamic	Muscle transposition: regional (temporalis, masseter, digastric) or free muscle neurovascular anastomosis (gracilis,and so forth)
4	Static	Suspension techniques (palmaris longus, fascia lata, gore-tex sling) or facial rejuvenation (face lift, brow lift, blepharoplasty)
5	Static	Eye care (gold weight, tarsorrhaphy, canthoplasty, dacryocystorhinostomy)
6	Static	Management of synkinesis (selective myectomy, neurectomy, Botox)

Data from Conley J, May M. Rehabilitation techniques for acute and long-standing facial paralysis. In: The facial nerve. May's 2nd edition. New York: Thieme; 2000. p. 562–9; with permission.

would not attempt a Group I or II surgery (*vide infra*) if the duration of paralysis exceeds 2 years or more. This algorithm may have developed on the unproven assumption that with long-term denervation the target muscles for reinnervation are atrophied. In fact, the obstruction to reinnervation could be a fibrosed distal nerve segment [8] or deposition of collagen on the basal lamina [6]. Currently, no tests exist to evaluate these structures noninvasively. Thus, attempts at reinnervation become empiric. Conley and colleagues [5] have reported successful outcomes in very late cases. The ideal procedure is one that would allow mimetic facial motion without synkinesis or additional neurologic deficit. Theoretically, the procedures described in Groups I and II could achieve these objectives in the authors' two cases. In the first case, if the opportunity had existed to obtain EMG studies even 3 years after the original injury, and if fibrillation potentials were still recorded, reinnervation surgery could have been offered to this patient. Surgery success would depend on accurate frozen section study of the segments of nerve proximal and distal to the area of the geniculate ganglion. If the proximal fibrotic segment extended deep into the internal auditory canal, anastomosis with an interpositional graft would be difficult technically, and in such a case a XII-VII jump graft would be most appropriate. If, despite this surgery, there was failure of reinnervation, the patient could have been offered free muscle graft and cross-facial anastomosis, particularly as he was so young. Unfortunately, the patient refused further investigations or surgery.

The second patient presents two problems: the residual meningioma and the long-term facial paralysis. It could be argued that the meningioma can be followed conservatively with serial MRI scans. If this course is taken, the preferred Group I procedure would not be possible, but the patient could benefit from a cross-over procedure such as a XII-VII jump graft, distal to the tumor. Given the patient's young age, the authors recommend tumor excision under frozen section control and restoration of the anatomic continuity of the nerve with an interpositional graft. Again, as in the previous case, if the tumor extends deep into the internal auditory canal, it will be excised under frozen section control and a XII-VII jump graft will be offered. If this fails as well, muscle transposition will be recommended, as in the previous case.

Summary

The preoperative evaluation for either revision facial nerve surgery or long-standing facial paralysis is far from comprehensive and typically is limited to an EMG assessment. The EMG can determine if fibrillation potentials are present; however, these do not necessarily indicate the degree of muscle viability. To the best of the authors' knowledge, no scientific correlation exists between EMG fibrillation potentials and either the degree of muscle atrophy, or the potential for a successful outcome of dynamic reanimation procedures. Clearly, controlled, double-blinded longitudinal study of chronic facial denervation and correlation with longitudinal EMG studies in the same cohort is needed.

References

[1] May M. Nerve repair. In: May M, Schaitkin BM, editors. The facial nerve. May's 2nd edition. New York: Thieme; 2000. p. 571–609.

[2] May M, Gantz B, Hughes G. Management of failed nerve graft following facial nerve resection for facial nerve neurofibroma. Head Neck Surg 1987;9:184–7.

[3] Kreutzberg GW, Raivich G. Neurobiology of regeneration and degeneration. In: May M, Schaitkin BM, editors. The facial nerve. May's 2nd edition. New York: Thieme; 2000. p. 67–79.

[4] Stennert E. Synkineses and the autoparalytic syndrome. In: Beurskens CHG, Van Gelder RS, Heymans PG, Manni JJ, Nicolai JA, editors. The facial palsies–complementary approaches. 1st edition. Utrecht, The Netherlands: Lemma Publishers; 2005. p. 117–33.

[5] Conley J, Hamaker RC, Donnenfeld H. Long-standing facial paralysis rehabilitation. Laryngoscope 1974;84:2155–62.

[6] Carlson BM. Skeletal muscle-denervation, reinnervation, and muscle transplantation. In: May M, Schaitkin BM, editors. The facial nerve. May's 2nd edition. New York: Thieme; 2000. p. 81–94.

[7] Felix H, Eby TL, Fisch U. New aspects of facial nerve pathology in temporal bone fractures. Acta Otolaryngol 1991;111:332–6.

[8] Ylikoski J, Hitselberger WE, House WF, et al. Degenerative changes in the distal stump of the severed human facial nerve. Acta Otolaryngol 1981;92:239–48.

[9] Belal A Jr. Structure of human muscle in facial paralysis. J Laryngol Otol 1982;96:325–34.

[10] Bardosi A. Schwann cell recruitment from intact nerve fibers. Exp Neurol 1989;103:123–34.

[11] Gagnon NB, Molina-Negro P. Facial reinnervation after facial paralysis: is it ever too late? Arch Otorhinolaryngol 1989;246:303–7.

[12] Chaudhry V, Cornblath DR. Wallerian degeneration in human nerves: serial electrophysiological studies. Muscle Nerve 1992;15:687–93.

[13] Kimura J. Electrodiagnosis in diseases of nerve and muscle: principles and practice. 3rd edition. New York: Oxford University Press; 2001.

[14] Aminoff M. In: Aminoff MJ, editor. Electromyography in clinical practice: clinical and electrodiagnostic aspects of neuromuscular disease. 3rd edition. New York: Churchill Livingstone; 1997. p. 67–8.

[15] Pribnow D, Johnson-Pais T, Bond CT, et al. Skeletal muscle and small-conductance calcium-activated potassium channels. Muscle Nerve 1999;22:742–50.

[16] Matar W, Lunde JA, Jasmin BJ, et al. Denervation enhances the physiological effects of the K(ATP) channel during fatigue in EDL and soleus muscle. Am J Physiol Regul Integr Comp Physiol 2001;281:R56–65.

[17] Brown W, Bolton C, MJ A. In: Aminoff MJ, editor. Neuromuscular function and disease. Philadelphia: W.B. Saunders; 2002. p. 354.

[18] Conley J, May M. Rehabilitation techniques for acute and long-standing facial paralysis. In: May M, Schaitkin BM, editors. The facial nerve. May's 2nd edition. New York: Thieme; 2000. p. 562–9.

Otolaryngol Clin N Am
39 (2006) 833–839

OTOLARYNGOLOGIC
CLINICS
OF NORTH AMERICA

Revision Cochlear Implantation

J. Thomas Roland Jr, MD*, Tina C. Huang, MD, Noel L. Cohen, MD

Department of Otolaryngology, New York University School of Medicine, 530 First Avenue, Suite 3C, New York, NY 10016, USA

Reoperation on a patient with an indwelling cochlear implant is uncommon. When necessary, surgery is performed for explantation of an existing device with immediate or delayed reimplantation, or for scalp flap revision and receiver-stimulator repositioning in the case of infection or device migration. Rarely, revision surgery is performed to reintroduce intracochlear electrodes that may have partly or entirely extruded from the cochlea or were placed inappropriately. Successful revision cochlear implant surgery requires attention to certain surgical principles. Good outcomes, as measured by speech perception tests, are common, but are not guaranteed. This article outlines the indications for revision cochlear implant surgery, the recommended surgical principles, and published outcomes from reimplantation.

Indications for revision or reimplantation

Device failure is the most common cause for revision cochlear implant surgery. Reimplantation is performed expeditiously, as usually the patient is rendered deaf by the device failure. This situation is usually very stressful for the patient. A common symptom of a hard failure is a lack of communication between the internal and external hardware, with no sound perception when the device is activated. Additional symptoms include abnormal sounds, painful sensations, and frequent or increased need for mapping. Confirming that the external hardware is functioning is the first step in a failure evaluation. Usually, voltage growth measurements, integrity testing, and radiographic analysis are performed in all cases where a lock between the internal and functioning external hardware is obtained, but abnormal sound percepts, painful sensations, and intermittency exist.

---

* Corresponding author.
E-mail address: tom.roland@med.nyu.edu (J.T. Roland).

0030-6665/06/$ - see front matter © 2006 Elsevier Inc. All rights reserved.
doi:10.1016/j.otc.2006.04.005

oto.theclinics.com

An increasing problem in cochlear implantation is the "soft" failure. In this condition, patients continue to derive some benefit from their devices. They often have a more prolonged failure prodrome and less obvious symptoms. In a recently published study, Waltzman and colleagues [1] found that 7 of 27 children who underwent reimplantation had documented performance decrement on routine perception testing, providing an early suspicion of a failing device. An increasing number of electrode short circuits or open circuits might also indicate an impending failure. The authors seriously consider reimplantation when more than three electrodes become "out of compliance." These patients are evaluated more regularly, and repeated integrity tests are performed. The timing of explantation and reimplantation depends on the type of symptoms the patient is having, patient preference, and the amount of performance reduction found on testing.

Receiver-stimulator migration is a rare complication and usually is prevented by surgically implanting the device in a bony well with secure suture fixation to bone. Suture fixation has always been a routine part of cochlear implantation in the authors' center. Allergic responses to the Silastic material, infection, and new bone growth are all causes of device migration. Revision scalp flap surgery is a treatment option, especially if no significant infection is present.

Electrode extrusion from the cochlea is uncommon [2]. It occurs more frequently in patients who had only partial insertions initially and in patients with known cochlear ossification. Reimplantation is considered when performance decrement is documented, but is often not indicated or necessary with the extrusion of only a few electrodes. Surveillance measures are increased when electrode extrusion is first detected. Serial plain film radiographs, more frequent mapping sessions, and more frequent performance testing assist the clinicians and patients with the revision surgery decision.

Infections, although less frequent, remain a common reason for revision cochlear implant surgery. An exposed, and therefore contaminated, device requires immediate attention and intervention, which includes culture-directed intravenous antibiotics and revision flap surgery. Significant scalp flap infections without device exposure also usually require surgical intervention with debridement, vigorous irrigation, and prolonged antibiotic therapy. Salvaging a device depends on the organism involved, the severity of the infection, and the presence of biofilms. Many investigators have reported successful revision flap surgery without removing a functioning device [3,4].

Surgical considerations

Reoperation for a failed or failing cochlear implant requires thoughtful planning and consideration of several issues. Most of the time, the same incision used for the first operation is opened and similar flaps are developed. It is important to avoid monopolar cautery to prevent current spread through the device to the delicate neural elements of the cochlea. Although this type of complication has never been documented, it could render an ear unsuitable for cochlear implantation. Additionally, current spread from the electrocautery might cause further damage to the internal receiver-stimulator's circuitry. The explanted device is returned routinely to the manufacturer for analysis and the information obtained is used in designing future devices. Electrical damage from cautery can confound this analysis. Several investigators have warned against the use of monopolar cautery, and even against bipolar cautery [5]. Roland and colleagues [6] have advocated the use of the Shaw heated scalpel that uses a sharp heated blade, and reported no wound healing delays or alopecia with its use. Laszig and colleagues [7] have advocated the use of the Ultracision harmonic scalpel that uses mechanical vibrations to cause denaturation of proteins from transfer of mechanical energy to the tissues. They also reported no wound healing difficulties.

During reoperation, mechanical damage to the explanted device should be avoided. The electrode lead wire might be encased in new bone and additional drilling and excavation is usually required. The intracochlear electrode is left in place until reimplantation is performed, either during the same surgical procedure or at a future date in the case of infection, and is accomplished by cutting the electrode at the facial recess or in the mastoid cavity. The electrode acts as a stent, keeping the intracochlear pseudocapsule open and preventing scalar occlusion by new bone growth in the case of delayed reimplantation. The manufacturers can still perform "cause-of-failure" analysis by reattaching the fine electrode wires in the laboratory.

In situations where the receiver-stimulator has migrated, or where a serious infection has occurred, usually the bed or well is also revised or relocated and new subcortical suture holes are made to secure the device. Care is taken not to dislodge the intra-cochlear electrodes. An intraoperative radiograph is recommended to confirm success. If the device has been exposed by scalp flap breakdown, the area is irrigated copiously with antibiotic-containing solution and the tissues around the device are debrided aggressively (Fig. 1). On occasion, when device salvage is attempted, a larger scalp flap may have to be designed to rotate healthy vascularized tissue over the device. When surgical salvage is unsuccessful, usually because of persistent or recurrent infection after 6 weeks of intravenous antibiotic therapy, the receiver-stimulator is removed, with the electrode array remaining in the cochlea. Three months of flap healing permits reimplantation in a sterile environment.

Electrode choice for revision surgery requires consideration. If many years have passed since the initial surgery, new device options will have become available. The new electrode should not be larger in diameter than the explanted electrode. Also, a reimplantation case may develop an obstructed cochlea situation requiring obstructed cochlea techniques. A split or double array device may be required, especially if there is significant luminal

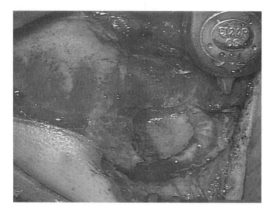

Fig. 1. Elevated scalp flap with old and new well delineated, and device held forward during a revision surgery for infection.

obstruction by ossification of the scala tympani, and should be available in the operating room; however, this situation is rare. Scala vestibuli insertions are considered if full insertion is not accomplished in the lower scala (Fig. 2) [8]. In patients with labyrinthitis ossificans, reimplantation can be even more challenging. Telian and colleagues [9] described two children who required revision of their implants after partial electrode insertion during the first surgery. They used a modified Rambo technique to access the cochlea, and the second turn of the cochlea was either opened or blue-lined. The basal turn was drilled out between the internal carotid artery and the second turn of the cochlea, and the electrode inserted. The first child, deafened

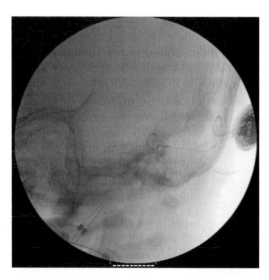

Fig. 2. Intraoperative fluoroscopic image of an electrode placed in a malformed cochlea.

postlingually, gained significant speech discrimination abilities, whereas the second child, deafened prelingually, achieved improved auditory awareness. The same device can be used for electrode extrusion, or a new device might be necessary. The authors have repositioned electrodes using the same device when the original electrodes were placed inadvertently in the internal auditory canal during the original operation. Intraoperative fluoroscopy provides real-time guidance for effective and successful intracochlear electrode placement (Fig. 3).

Outcomes

The first reports of cochlear reimplantation were published in the 1980s. In 1985, Hochmair-Desoyer and Burian [10] described two subjects who underwent reimplantation for gradual device failure. Scar tissue and new bone formation were encountered during the surgery, but new electrodes were inserted without difficulty, and thresholds and speech performance were stable postreimplantation. Jackler and colleagues [11] published a cat model of a large series of subjects implanted with different makes of implants who required revision and reimplantation. Electrode placement within the cochlea was successful in most subjects, although scar and granulation tissue was noted around the scala tympani, round window, facial recess, and middle ear. The subjects with difficult reinsertions often had increased granulation tissue, which was associated with Gelfoam use in the animal experiments. The investigators described a fibrous envelope around the electrode within the scala tympani and osteoanagenesis within the scala tympani. They were the first to suggest cutting the electrode array at the round window and leaving it within the scala tympani as a lumen retainer in cases of delayed reimplantation secondary to collapse of the fibrous capsule. Their animal studies showed that, although reimplantation was feasible, there was a twofold increase in traumatic insertions. Most of the subjects achieved functional results. In addition to the fibrous capsule around the electrode array within the scala tympani, Woolford, Saeed, and colleagues [12,13] reported on a fibrous capsule around the receiver-stimulator, granulation tissue and fibrosis around the electrode within the mastoid bowl, and new bone growth around the subcortical channel for the proximal electrode array. Their subjects also showed stable or improved performance after reimplantation.

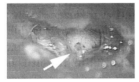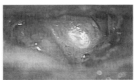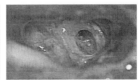

Fig. 3. View through facial recess with obstructed scala tympani and new cochleostomy in a patent scala vestibule. Obstructed previously operated scala tympani (*arrow*).

In 1996, Parisier and colleagues [14] reported a 14.9% pediatric failure rate, as compared with the national pediatric failure rate of approximately 9%, whereas their adult failure rate was 2%, comparable to the 2.5% national adult failure rate. Their findings at revision surgery were similar to those reported previously. They used only bipolar cautery until the old device was explanted, and suggested preserving the mastoid-cranial periosteum as a separate layer for use as an additional flap, and avoiding the modiolar area to decrease the risk of a cerebrospinal fluid leak. They were able to reinsert every electrode array after removing the fibrous and bony overgrowths without complications, and performance level was the same or improved after reimplantation. By 1998, 5-year failure rates for the Cochlear Corporation and Advanced Bionics were estimated to be less than 1.5%. Balkany and colleagues [15] reported a failure rate of 5.7%. They had no complications in their series of revision implants, and again found ossification of the cochleostomy, mastoid fibrosis, and fibrous or bony obstruction of the scala tympani. Their subjects performed at least as well as before revision and they achieved a significantly longer insertion length at revision surgery. Conversely, Miyamoto and colleagues [16] found a statistically shorter insertion length at revision and a significantly reduced number of clinically useful active channels.

Current reports on reimplantation performance uniformly report equal or improved performance for both adults and children. Alexiades and colleagues [17] found that adults who received the same device showed a significant performance benefit, whereas those who received an upgraded device showed no improvement. Parisier and colleagues' report [18] on pediatric revision implants found that the speech perception scores of all their children were either the same or improved after reimplantation, with 68% achieving open-set speech recognition. A later report by the same group [19] confirmed their pediatric findings. Again, mention was made of the universal finding of varying degrees of ossification around the cochleostomy. Hamzavi and colleagues [20], using the Med-El Combi 40 + device, found no statistically significant difference in their subjects' overall performance after reimplantation, although there was a significant improvement in the Innsbrucker Sentence Test scores. Lassig and colleagues [21] found that 71.4% of their subjects had improved speech recognition, 20% showed little or no change, and 8.5% had decreased performance. The one subject who showed significant decrease in performance experienced device failure and was reimplanted with an upgraded device.

Initial reports describe reimplantation caused by device failure or hard failures. However, devices are being explanted for soft failures as well. Buchman and colleagues [22] found that 87% of subjects reimplanted for soft failures had improved auditory ability and 91% had resolution of their non-auditory symptoms. Their subjects also showed a significant improvement in speech understanding.

Revision cochlear implant surgery, although uncommon, presents the clinician with several challenges. Thoughtful preparation and patient counseling, combined with appropriate procedures, will lead to successful outcomes in most cases. The patient should be aware that a reimplantation, even with a newer generation of device, will not always lead to improved outcomes.

References

[1] Waltzman SB, Roland JT, Waltzman M, et al. Cochlear reimplantation in children: soft signs, symptoms and results. Cochlear Implants Int 2004;5(4):138–45.

[2] Roland JT, Fishman AJ, Waltzman SB, et al. Stability of the cochlear implant array in children. Laryngoscope 1998;108(8):1119–23.

[3] Antonelli PJ, Lee JC, Burne RA. Bacterial biofilms may contribute to persistent cochlear implant infection. Otol Neurotol 2004;25(6):953–7.

[4] Rubinstein JT, Gantz BJ, Parkinson WS. Management of cochlear implant infections. Am J Otol 1999;20(1):46–9.

[5] Handoussa A. Cochlear reimplantation. Adv Otorhinolaryngol 2000;57:123–6.

[6] Roland JT Jr, Fishman AJ, Waltzman SB, et al. The Shaw scalpel in revision cochlear implant surgery. Ann Otol Rhinol Laryngol Suppl 2000;185:23–5.

[7] Laszig R, Ridder GJ, Aschendorff A, et al. Ultracision: an alternative to electrocautery in revision cochlear implant surgery. Laryngoscope 2002;112:190–1.

[8] Marrinan M, Roland JT, Lin K. Intentional scala vestibuli cochlear implant electrode insertion. Otol Neurotol, in press.

[9] Telian SA, Zimmerman-Phillips S, Kileny PR. Successful revision of failed cochlear implants in severe labyrinthitis ossificans. Am J Otol 1996;17:53–60.

[10] Hochmair-Desoyer IJ, Burian K. Reimplantation of a molded scala tympani electrode: impact on psychophysical and speech discrimination abilities. Ann Otol Rhinol Laryngol 1985; 94:65–70.

[11] Jackler RK, Leake PA, McKerrow WS. Cochlear implant revision: effects of reimplantation on the cochlea. Ann Otol Rhinol Laryngol 1989;98:813–20.

[12] Woolford TJ, Saeed SR, Boyd P, et al. Cochlear reimplantation. Ann Otol Rhinol Laryngol Suppl 1995;166:449–53.

[13] Saeed SR, Ramsden RT, Hartley C, et al. Cochlear reimplantation. J Laryngol Otol 1995; 109:980–5.

[14] Parisier SC, Chute PM, Popp AL. Cochlear implant mechanical failures. Am J Otol 1996;17: 730–4.

[15] Balkany TJ, Hodges AV, Gomez-Marin O, et al. Cochlear reimplantation. Laryngoscope 1999;109(3):351–5.

[16] Miyamoto RT, Svirsky MA, Myres WA, et al. Cochlear implant reimplantation. Am J Otol 1997;18:S60–1.

[17] Alexiades G, Roland JT Jr, Fishman AJ, et al. Cochlear reimplantation: surgical techniques and functional results. Laryngoscope 2001;111:1608–13.

[18] Parisier SC, Chute PM, Popp AL, et al. Outcome analysis of cochlear implant reimplantation in children. Laryngoscope 2001;111:26–32.

[19] Fayad JN, Baino T, Parisier SC. Revision cochlear implant surgery: causes and outcome. Otolaryngol Head Neck Surg 2004;131:429–32.

[20] Hamzavi J, Baumgartner WD, Pok SM. Does cochlear reimplantation affect speech recognition? Int J Audiol 2002;41:151–6.

[21] Lassig A, Zwolan TA, Telian SA. Cochlear implant failures and revision. Otol Neurotol 2005;26:624–34.

[22] Buchman CA, Higgins CA, Cullen R, et al. Revision cochlear implant surgery in adult patients with suspected device malfunction. Otol Neurotol 2004;25:504–10.

ELSEVIER
SAUNDERS

Otolaryngol Clin N Am
39 (2006) 841–844

OTOLARYNGOLOGIC
CLINICS
OF NORTH AMERICA

Index

Note: Page numbers of article titles are in **boldface** type.

0030-6665/06/$ - see front matter © 2006 Elsevier Inc. All rights reserved.
doi:10.1016/S0030-6665(06)00098-3

oto.theclinics.com